The
ABC of
CBT

SAGE was founded in 1965 by Sara Miller McCune to support the dissemination of usable knowledge by publishing innovative and high-quality research and teaching content. Today, we publish over 900 journals, including those of more than 400 learned societies, more than 800 new books per year, and a growing range of library products including archives, data, case studies, reports, and video. SAGE remains majority-owned by our founder, and after Sara's lifetime will become owned by a charitable trust that secures our continued independence.

Los Angeles | London | New Delhi | Singapore | Washington DC | Melbourne

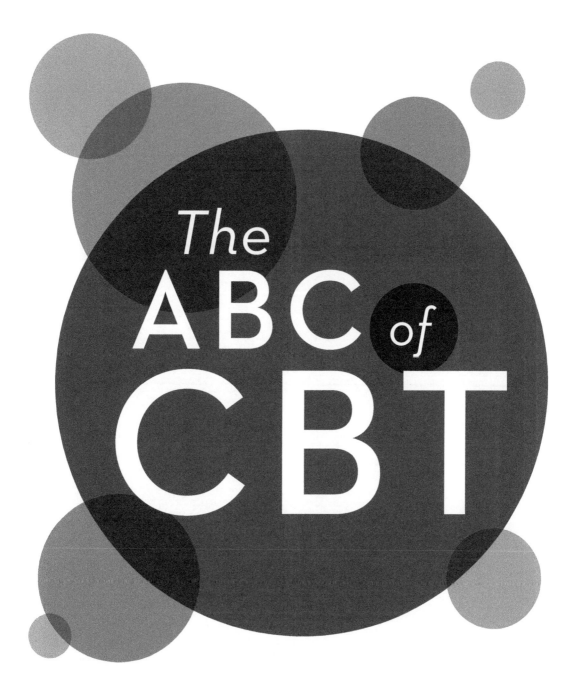

The ABC of CBT

HELEN KENNERLEY

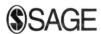

Los Angeles | London | New Delhi
Singapore | Washington DC | Melbourne

To my family, of course.

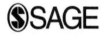

Los Angeles | London | New Delhi
Singapore | Washington DC | Melbourne

SAGE Publications Ltd
1 Oliver's Yard
55 City Road
London EC1Y 1SP

SAGE Publications Inc.
2455 Teller Road
Thousand Oaks, California 91320

SAGE Publications India Pvt Ltd
B 1/I 1 Mohan Cooperative Industrial Area
Mathura Road
New Delhi 110 044

SAGE Publications Asia-Pacific Pte Ltd
3 Church Street
#10-04 Samsung Hub
Singapore 049483

Editor: Susannah Trefgarne
Assistant editor: Ruth Lilly
Production editor: Rachel Burrows
Copyeditor: Aud Scriven
Proofreader: Genevieve Friar
Indexer: Gary Kirby
Marketing manager: Dilhara Attygalle
Cover design: Naomi Robinson
Typeset by: Cenveo Publisher Services
Printed in the UK

Library of Congress Control Number: 2020937758

British Library Cataloguing in Publication data

A catalogue record for this book is available from the British Library

ISBN 978-1-5264-9133-6
ISBN 978-1-5264-9132-9 (pbk)

At SAGE we take sustainability seriously. Most of our products are printed in the UK using responsibly sourced papers and boards. When we print overseas we ensure sustainable papers are used as measured by the PREPS grading system. We undertake an annual audit to monitor our sustainability.

CONTENTS

ABOUT THE AUTHOR

Helen Kennerley, DPhil, is a Consultant Clinical Psychologist and founding fellow of the Oxford Cognitive Therapy Centre (OCTC), where she was for many years Director of the postgraduate courses in Advanced Cognitive Therapy Studies and the MSc in Cognitive Behavioural Therapy. She is currently the lead for the OCTC/University of Oxford Post-graduate Certificates in Supervision and Training and in Psychological Trauma. She is also a Consultant Clinical Psychologist with the MOD. She has made valuable contributions to the field of cognitive therapy through her popular workshops and her writings. Among other publications, she is the author of *Overcoming Anxiety* and co-author of *An Introduction to Cognitive Behaviour Therapy*, both of which have been highly commended by the British Medical Association. In 2002, Helen was also voted one of the most influential female cognitive therapists in Britain by BABCP members.

PREFACE

This book is a brief guide to Beckian CBT, the psychotherapy developed by Aaron T. Beck over forty years ago. It will sit amongst several other CBT texts and you might be wondering what makes this one worth reading.

One reason is its brevity and another is its comprehensiveness. My aim is to offer a coherent overview of CBT and if it piques your interest, it will have provided you with a foundation for more fully developing your understanding and skill by reading some of the lengthier texts. It's a CBT primer if you like.

Essentially, it has four sections:

1. An introduction to CBT (Chapter 1)
2. Building a foundation for CBT (Chapters 2–6)
3. The techniques of CBT (Chapters 7–9)
4. Taking things forward (Chapter 10 and the worksheets)

Each section takes a transdiagnostic approach so you will be learning about the application of CBT across disorders and you will see just how versatile an intervention it is.

This brief guide owes a lot to a longer text, *An Introduction to Cognitive Behaviour Therapy: Skills and Applications*, which was jointly written by Joan Kirk, David Westbrook and me back in 2007. Writing that first edition and then reviewing the content for later editions enabled us to refine as well as update our thinking, and I believe that the content of this *ABC of CBT* reflects a good deal of the thinking of two great CBT therapists, Joan and David. Another good reason to read this book.

ACKNOWLEDGEMENTS

First, always first, I must thank the patients who over the years have helped deepen my appreciation of CBT. Without their openness and courage to embark on a therapeutic journey this text would be just theoretical rambling.

Then thanks are owed to the tutors, mentors, supervisees and students who have guided my training and fueled my learning. Sometimes this has been formally but in Oxford I have been exposed to the most wonderful informal education over many years. On my first day in the Department of Psychiatry, in 1980, John Teasdale chatted with me about his cognitive research and within a few days I took part in one of David Clark's trials and then sat with him talking about his investigations over a drink. My recreational education continued with Liz Campbell and Peter Cooper's inspirational hosting: I developed my enthusiasm for CBT over supper at their homes. Anyone in the Oxford Department of Psychiatry at that time will remember the very important coffee breaks where we clustered round a hissing, puffing coffee machine and then chatted about theory, research and sometimes celebrity gossip. Vivid in my memory are Gillian Butler, Pepe Catalan, June Dent, Keith Hawton, Anne Hackmann, Derek Johnson, Paul Salkovskis, to name but a few who shaped my perceptions of CBT. For me Melanie Fennel was a particularly important member of this crowd because she gave me one-to-one training in CBT. What a privilege. And I owe a real debt to Joan Kirk who gave me my first CBT post. She was also one of the best scientist-practitioner models one could ever imagine. Later still, more inspirational cognitive therapists joined the department, each taking CBT in new directions and each influencing my take on its contemporary use: Anke Elhers, Emily Holmes, Freda McManus, Kate Muse, Sarah Rakovshik, Roz Safran, Mark Williams, again just to name a few. Each brought exciting new thinking about both cognitive theory and its practice – creative and diverse thinking. And Oxford drew 'big names' who gave talks or spent sabbaticals here – so we mixed and mingled with the likes of Aaron T. Beck himself, Kate Davidson, Mark Freeston, Paul Gilbert, Kathleen Mooney, Stirling Moorey, Christine Padesky, Jan Scott, Glenn Waller – all of whom have left traces of their wisdom. And when I moved from the University to the NHS department, there were more inspiring colleagues. In particular, the late David Westbrook, with whom I was able to write and rigorously refine my thinking about CBT practice. I'm also very grateful to colleagues with whom I've collaborated in teaching CBT basics: discussions around these OCTC workshops have been so important in refining my view of CBT.

Although this might sound like an exercise in name dropping, it is a reminder that underpinning this CBT primer is a very rich and dynamic four-decade foundation. I was fortunate to be working in a world actively steeped in CBT over that time and I hope that this is communicated in *The ABC of CBT* so that it offers more than a snapshot of CBT. I hope that it gives you the context of its development and a vision of where you might take it.

Last, and when I say 'not least' I mean it, I want to thank the staff at SAGE who asked me to write this book, guided me through the early stages, were patient in the latter stages and who throw the best professional party ever.

Helen Kennerley
Oxford, 2020

1

WHAT IS CBT?

The form of cognitive therapy described in this book is cognitive behaviour therapy (CBT), a talking therapy pioneered by Dr A.T. Beck in Philadelphia in the 1970s.

CBT helps people manage problems by helping them change the way they think and behave, which in turn changes the way they *feel*. That's the goal of CBT, changing the way we feel, because *feeling* more confident, or less distressed, or less miserable is what makes the difference.

Beck's background was in neurology and psychodynamic psychotherapy, but in the 1960s and 1970s he drew on contemporary behaviour therapy and the emerging cognitive therapies in developing his own version of a cognitive-behavioural psychotherapy for depression. Treatment trials of CBT (e.g. Rush, Beck, Kovacs & Hollon, 1977) showed that it was an effective intervention for depression, and the first treatment manual, *Cognitive Therapy of Depression*, was published by Beck and his colleagues in 1979. This is still my go-to text, and if you haven't read it I would recommend that you do so. There is no better foundation for a practising CBT therapist because it captures the essence of Beckian CBT – practical guidelines combined with Beck's vision and philosophy. You might be interested to learn that the second chapter in the book focuses on the role of emotions in CBT and the third chapter is devoted to the therapeutic relationship. This immediately challenges the myths that CBT does not attend to feelings and that it disregards the therapeutic alliance.

There are also other myths about CBT that the book corrects, for example that CBT is a rather simple 'cookbook' approach to therapy – if a person has *this* problem then we use *that* technique. CBT is so much more than a mechanical application of techniques: it hinges on understanding a patient's problem, understanding CBT theory, and then bringing the two together in a formulation that is particular to that patient and will then guide therapy (see Chapter 5).

Another myth is that CBT is about positive thinking, but it's actually about developing a realistic outlook, keeping fears or misery or anger in proportion. And if there is a real problem to be addressed then the CBT shifts to problem-solving.

Beck's CBT rapidly developed as a successful intervention not only for depression but also for a range of anxiety disorders, anger problems, trauma-related problems, eating disorders, relationship difficulties and many other psychological and medical issues. It has stood the test of time by maintaining a very respectable research foundation. It was partly this compelling empirical support for CBT that led to it being central to the government's Improving Access to Psychological Therapies (IAPT: see www.iapt.nhs.uk) programme in 2008. IAPT has resulted in a year-on-year increase in the provision of CBT within the NHS in England and Wales with the aim of training over ten thousand therapists by 2021. The impact of IAPT has been rigorously evaluated and preliminary data from the pilot sites supported the effectiveness of the programme (Clark, 2018).

THE CBT APPROACH

The approach adopted in CBT is distinguished by a combination of characteristics that will be elaborated later in this text, but in order to set the scene here's a summary.

- The relationship between patient and therapist is collaborative: it's a working partnership.
- The therapy itself is overt, structured and active.
- Therapy is time-limited and (usually) brief.
- The approach of both therapist and patient is empirical.
- CBT is essentially problem-oriented.

A collection of basic principles also defines CBT. You'll see that several of them apply to other forms of psychological intervention, but it's the way that they are brought together that forms the foundation of modern CBT.

1. The cognitive principle

To illustrate a point when teaching, my former colleague, David Westbrook, would sometimes quote Hamlet in conversation with Rosencrantz: 'there is nothing either good or bad, but thinking makes it so.' The point it illustrates is key to CBT, namely that emotional reactions are strongly influenced by *cognitions*. By cognition we mean thoughts, mental images, beliefs and interpretations – the *meaning* we make of our experiences.

This is illustrated by the simple example of two people losing their jobs.

The first person is miserable, and it is easy to assume that he's down because he has lost his job. This may be true – that the job loss caused depression. However, the second person is quite jolly so it can't be as simple as 'job loss causes depression'. We need to find out what this particular life event *meant* to the individual.

The first man's thoughts were along the lines of: 'This is terrible. I'm going to struggle to get another job at my age and I still have bills to pay.' This would certainly make sense of his misery. In contrast, the second man felt relieved when he was fired because he'd been anguishing over what to do as he was unhappy at work. Now he had some compensation money to tide him over while he pursued something that suited him better, and he'd been spared the stress of making the decision to resign.

Now imagine another scenario: Anita is at a party where no-one immediately speaks to her. She could interpret this in many ways and she could experience different emotions:

- 'I can't think of anything to say to anyone. I will look so boring and stupid.' [This could lead to anxiety]
- 'No surprise here. Nobody ever wants to talk to me, people just don't like me.' [Which could have a depressing outcome]
- 'People are so snooty. Who do these guests think they are?' [A response that might trigger anger]
- 'Typical party, everyone's got someone to chat with. I guess it's up to me to make the first move.' [This reaction might even result in some anticipatory excitement]

Again we see that the meaning that we make of an event matters. This explains why not everyone is brought down by a relationship break-up or the diagnosis of an illness, just as not everyone is elated when they win a lottery or get a promotion. When two people react differently to an event it is because they are seeing it differently. The way they view it will affect their feelings and this in turn can influence their *behaviour*.

2. The behavioural principle

CBT also considers that what we *do* (our behaviour) can be crucial in maintaining or in changing our psychological states. Consider the above example again.

Anita's behaviour could have a significant effect on her thoughts and feelings. For example, if she approached another guest and chatted she might discover that the guest was friendly, and as a result she may be less inclined to think negatively about people in the future. On the other hand, if she withdrew and avoided joining the party she would not have a chance to find out if her thoughts were accurate or not, and her negative thoughts and feelings might persist. She might then be less inclined to accept the next social invitation.

Thus, CBT presumes that behaviour can have a strong impact on thoughts and emotions, and in particular that changing what a person *does* is often a powerful way of influencing thoughts and emotions.

3. The 'interacting systems' principle

CBT goes beyond just considering the way we feel or think or behave, it takes the view that experiences are interactions between various 'systems' within the person and in their environment:

- Cognition.
- Affect or Emotion.
- Behaviour.
- Physiology.

These systems interact not only with each other but also with the environment (i.e. the physical, social, family, cultural and economic environment). Figure 1.1, based on Padesky and Mooney's five-system framework (Padesky & Mooney, 1990), illustrates the way in which the systems impact on each other so that change in one can affect the entire framework.

Hence a shift in cognitions can influence emotions, sensations or behaviour and vice versa, and in addition the individual impacts on the environment and vice versa. It is important that we take this dynamic feature into account when we assess a person's problems. If we don't grasp this interacting and bigger picture, then we risk missing something that could be crucial to understanding why a problem isn't going away. This will be explored more in Chapters 5 and 6 when we look at formulation and assessment.

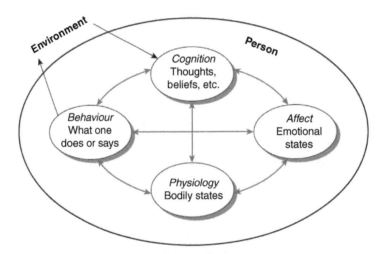

Figure 1.1 Interacting systems (Padesky & Mooney, 1990)

Source: 5-part model adapted with permission of the author, copyright 1986 by the Center for Cognitive Therapy; www.padesky.com

4. The 'working with what we see' principle

The main focus of therapy for the CBT therapist is on what is happening in the present, and what the patient shares overtly. The main concerns are with the processes currently maintaining the problem and so we focus on these, trying to break unhelpful patterns of cognition and behaviour. Having said this, CBT does not dismiss the past – far from it. In developing an understanding of the origin of a problem we review historical factors and Chapters 5 and 6 explore this further. Nor does CBT dismiss processes that might not yet be fully conscious. We do consider factors that might be outside our patient's awareness, but rather than developing an interpretation that is shared, we build a hypothesis and then check out our therapeutic hunch with the patient, usually using Socratic methods (which we will review in Chapters 7 and 8).

5. The empirical principle

CBT believes we should evaluate our practice as rigorously as possible, using data rather than just clinical anecdote or intuition. This is achieved in a number of ways:

> We refer to the outcomes of research trials in choosing our interventions so that our treatments are founded on tested and proven theories.

> Within a course of treatment, we regularly collect data in the form of mood and behaviour questionnaires, distress and confidence ratings and so on, so that we can evaluate the impact of the therapy.

> We develop hypotheses about our patients' problems and then set up experiments to test these out. We also teach our patients to do this for themselves.

In this way we operate as 'scientist-practitioners', identifying patterns, developing hunches, testing them out, and evaluating our progress. This might sound rather detached, but CBT is not a cool impersonal set of procedures, it's a therapy that takes place in the context of a supportive, empathic relationship – which brings us on to the next principle.

6. The interpersonal principle

In CBT Beck refers to the therapeutic relationship as the *working alliance*. CBT is not 'done to' a patient, instead we foster a milieu that enables us to work with a person, who engages with their full knowledge and consent. This is such an important principle that the next chapter is pretty much dedicated to it – so more later.

CBT COMPETENCES

A useful resource for any CBT therapist is the *CBT competences framework*, an initiative funded by the UK Department of Health, with the goal of identifying the necessary skills for providing good-quality CBT for anxiety and depression (Roth & Pilling, 2007). Roth and Pilling examined treatment manuals for effective CBT interventions for different disorders and produced a 'map' of competences divided into five domains:

- *Generic competences in psychological therapy.* These are the basic capabilities needed by a therapist from *any* school of therapy: e.g. knowledge of mental health, ability to relate to clients, and so on.
- *Basic CBT competences.* Skills related to the basic structure of CBT therapies, such as agenda-setting or use of homework.
- *Specific CBT techniques.* The core treatment strategies, such as using thought records and identifying and testing cognitions and beliefs.
- *Problem-specific competences.* Approaches used in treatment programmes for particular disorders, such as Beckian cognitive therapy for depression, or exposure and response prevention for obsessive-compulsive disorder.
- *Meta-competences.* The 'higher-level' skills that allow a therapist to make effective judgements about when to use which specific treatment strategy. Includes using the formulation to adapt treatment to an individual, dealing with difficulties during treatment, etc.

This book will address basic CBT competencies and specific techniques, but do go to the original Roth and Pilling (2007) publication for more detailed information about the entire competence framework.

IS CBT EFFECTIVE?

Given that we've raised CBT's commitment to empiricism it is reasonable to ask: what is the evidence that CBT is effective?

Evidence regarding CBT treatment

Since its inception, CBT has been subject to systematic evaluation and so we do have a sense of its clinical relevance. Roth and Fonagy (2005), in *What works for whom?*, report evidence showing that CBT is a strongly supported therapy for most adult psychological disorders, and has more support in more kinds of problem than any other therapy.

A second useful source of evidence is the UK National Institute for Health and Clinical Excellence (NICE). This is a government agency that surveys the evidence for the effectiveness of different treatments and makes recommendations about which treatments ought therefore to be made available in the National Health Service (NHS). Its guidelines on mental health conditions are periodically updated and so it is wise to visit the actual NICE website at www.nice.org.uk/guidance/conditions-and-diseases/mental-health-and-behavioural-conditions.

NICE has produced guidelines on several major mental-health problems, which include recommendations for offering CBT for Depression, Panic Disorder, Social Anxiety Disorder, Generalised Anxiety Disorder (GAD), Post-Traumatic Stress Disorder (PTSD), Obsessive Compulsive Disorder (OCD), Psychosis and Schizophrenia, and Eating Disorders. NICE also recommends CBT in the management of other conditions such as chronic fatigue syndrome, alcohol-use disorders, antenatal and postnatal mental-health problems.

So, in response to the question 'Is CBT effective?', CBT does display a solid and wide evidence base for efficacy and effectiveness, although of course there is always room for further evaluation.

LEVELS OF COGNITION

By now you will have a good idea what CBT looks like: it's an overt, active and structured therapy that brings about emotional (and behavioural) change by targeting cognitions. Our next step is exploring what we mean by *cognition*.

When we talk of cognitions, we refer not only to thoughts – which can readily be put into words – but also to images. Confusingly, in CBT we often use the term *thought*, as in *negative automatic thought* for example, even when we intend to include images. Not ideal, but it is the convention.

CBT distinguishes different levels of cognition. Various CBT practitioners might categorise cognitions slightly differently, but the following classification is commonly used:

- Automatic thoughts: a stream of cognitions that is usually readily accessible.
- Underlying assumptions: rules for living, predictions, expectations.
- Core beliefs: fundamental beliefs about ourselves, our world and our future.

In CBT we aim to focus on the Automatic Thoughts (ATs) rather than core beliefs, but because ATs are so influenced by core beliefs we will start there.

Core beliefs

This level of cognition is often referred to as the soil from which assumptions and automatic thoughts grow. In his early writings Beck referred to 'the cognitive triad' of core beliefs:

1. Self (*I am* ...).
2. The world (the world is ... or others are ...).
3. The future (the *future is* ...).

These represent fundamental views that influence mood and shape behaviours.

A person with depression would often have a view of self as unworthy or flawed, would consider the world unfair and the future hopeless. Someone with anxieties might see themselves as vulnerable to harm, the world as threatening and the future as unpredictable.

These fundamental views would make sense of the first person's depression and inactivity, while the perspective of the second person would explain anxiety and avoidance.

Typically core beliefs are:

- not immediately accessible to consciousness: they may have to be inferred by observation of characteristic thoughts and behaviours in many different situations;
- expressed as general and absolute statements, e.g. 'I am bad' or 'Others are not to be trusted': they tend not to vary much across times or situations but are experienced as fundamental truths that apply in all situations;
- usually developed early on in life as a result of childhood experiences, but they may sometimes emerge or change later in life, e.g. as a result of adult trauma.

Despite the potentially powerful impact of core beliefs we tend not to focus on these directly in short-term therapy. This is partly because they are usually not easy to capture and address, but also because they very often modify spontaneously when we address automatic thoughts and underlying assumptions. Therefore working at the level of ATs and UAs (Underlying Assumptions) can be sufficient to change core beliefs.

Yet another myth about CBT is that, by not focusing on fundamental core beliefs, the therapy is superficial and likely to result in relapse. It is easy to assume that core beliefs are at the root of the problem, or are the underlying cause, and therefore they must be tackled directly for therapy to be effective. However, most successful CBT research to date targets ATs, but that does not make the therapy ineffective or short-lived. This is probably for two reasons:

Reviewing and building evidence that tests ATs can have an impact, a 'knock-on effect' on core beliefs, so we don't need to target core beliefs directly.

People with common mental-health problems have a *range* of core beliefs, not just negative and unhelpful ones. Through the process of therapy, they can bring their more positive or functional beliefs back into operation and restore a functional balance.

Although there is not yet much research evidence, working directly with core beliefs may be more important in lifelong problems such as very chronic difficulties and personality disorders, where a person may never have formed much in the way of counter-balancing functional beliefs or the unhelpful beliefs may be very fixed.

Often a child or young person evolves negative core belief(s) followed by a way of dealing with that perspective, for example: *I am flawed and others are hurtful – but if I please everyone and keep out of trouble no-one will hurt me*. This way of coping might help them for a while, it might even protect them, but it would leave the core beliefs unchallenged. In adulthood there might be little to support the original core beliefs, but because of their longstanding and unchallenged status they might be very resistant to change. In such instances, a therapist might well need to target core beliefs and there are CBT guides to help us do this (e.g. Beck, Davis & Freeman, 2016; Davidson, Livingstone, McArthur, Dickson & Gumley, 2007).

Underlying assumptions

UAs can be considered as bridging the gap between core beliefs and ATs. They develop as a response to the core belief and are referred to as dysfunctional assumptions (DAs) when they backfire and hinder rather than help a person.

Core beliefs give us fundamental (and often thematic) perspectives whilst UAs can be thought of as 'rules for living', i.e. more specific in their applicability than core beliefs, but more general than ATs. They often take the form of conditional 'If … then … ' propositions, or they are framed as 'should' or 'must' statements. UAs often represent attempts to live with painful or frightening core beliefs. For example, if I believe that I am fundamentally unlovable, I may develop the assumption that:

- 'If I always try to please other people then they will tolerate me, but if I stand up for my own needs I will be rejected,' or
- 'If I keep a low profile, no-one will see the real me and never know that I am unlovable,' or
- 'I must always put other people's needs first, otherwise they will reject me.'

Such UAs offer hope that I can contain the situation and provide a guide to how to live my life so as to overcome some of the effects of the core belief, but it is always a fragile truce: if I fail to please someone, then I am in trouble. When one of my UAs is violated, then negative automatic thoughts (NATs) and strong emotions are likely to be triggered.

Characteristics of UAs are as follows:

- Like core beliefs, they are not as obvious as ATs and may not be easily verbalised. They often have to be inferred from actions or from patterns of common ATs.
- They are usually conditional statements, taking the form of 'If … then … ', or 'should/ must … otherwise …' statements. This makes them very amenable to behavioural testing.
- Some may be culturally reinforced, e.g. beliefs about putting others first, or the importance of success, may be approved of in some cultures.
- They become 'dysfunctional' when they are too rigid and over-generalised, not flexible enough to cope with the inevitable complications and setbacks of life.
- They are usually tackled later in therapy, after the patient has developed some ability to work with ATs. It is thought that modifying UAs may be helpful in developing resistance to relapse (Beck, Rush, Shaw & Emery, 1979).

Automatic thoughts (ATs)

These are the stream of thoughts (or images) that almost all of us can notice if we try to pay attention to them. They can be positive, neutral or negative in content. Negative automatic thoughts (NATs), as first described by Beck in his work with depressed patients, are often central to problems. These are negatively-tinged appraisals or interpretations – *meanings* we take from what happens around us or within us.

If you were to recall a recent time when you became upset and if you tried to remember what was going through your mind at that time you could probably pick out some NATs. For example, if you were anxious you might have had thoughts about the threat of something bad happening to you ('Oh no – now I'm messing up … ') or people you care about ('He's not going to manage this alone … '); if you were annoyed, you might have had thoughts about others being unfair, or not following rules you consider important ('Come on – that's so out of order!'); and if you were fed up, there might have been thoughts about loss or defeat, or negative views of yourself ('Here I go again – there's just no point … ').

ATs (and therefore NATs) are thought to exert a direct influence over mood from moment to moment, and they are thus of central importance to CBT. They have several common characteristics:

- As the name suggests, one does not have to *try* to think ATs – they just happen, automatically and without effort (although it may take effort to pay attention to them and notice them).
- They are specific thoughts about specific events or situations. Although they may become stereotyped, particularly in chronic problems, they may also vary a great deal from time to time and situation to situation.
- They are, or can easily become, conscious. Most people are either aware of this kind of thought, or can soon learn to be aware of them with some practice in self-monitoring.
- They may be so brief and frequent, so habitual, that they are not 'heard'. They are so much a part of our ordinary mental environment that unless we focus on them we may not notice them, any more than we notice breathing most of the time.
- They are often plausible and taken as obviously true, especially when emotions are strong. We tend not to question them: if I think 'I am useless' when I am feeling fed up about something having gone wrong, it seems a simple statement of the truth. One of the crucial steps in therapy is to help patients stop accepting their ATs in this way, but instead to step back and consider their accuracy. As a common CBT motto has it, 'Thoughts are opinions not facts' – and like all opinions they may or may not be accurate.
- Although we usually talk about ATs as if they were verbal constructs – e.g. 'I'm making a mess of this' – it is important to be aware that they may take the form of images. For example, in social phobia, rather than thinking in words, 'Other people think I'm peculiar', a person may get a mental image of themself looking red-faced, sweaty and incoherent.
- Because of their immediate effect on emotional states, and their accessibility, ATs are usually tackled early on in therapy. ATs are a therapist's first port of call cognitively speaking. This is where we start the CBT work.

You can see how these three levels of cognition relate to each other in Figure 1.2.

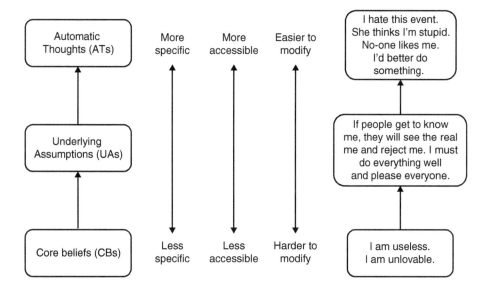

Figure 1.2 Illustration of levels of cognition

Cognitive processes

As well as considering the *content* of a person's thinking, we also look for unhelpful cognitive *processes* that can contribute to problems. This is the sort of thinking style that makes a person feel worse because it is:

- **Exaggerated** – only seeing the extremes of a situation or holding unrealistic standards or leaping to the very, very worst conclusion: *'This is terrible, everything always goes wrong.'*
- **Self-reproachful** – a person might be hard on themself, perhaps name-calling, taking things personally, all of which tends to make anyone feel even worse: *'Idiot – I'm so stupid!'*
- **Skewed towards the negative** – assuming the worst because of one event, or always seeing the glass as 'half empty', or dismissing positive experiences: *'I got that wrong – I'm useless at everything.'*
- **Based on intuition** – assuming that something must be true because it 'feels' true so there's no arguing with it, and this includes jumping to conclusions or 'mind-reading': *'I just know that I won't cope/that they think I'm a fool/that it's going to turn out badly.'*

Because of the interaction of thoughts, emotions and behaviour, extreme thinking tends to trigger extreme feelings and behaviours – and can so easily fuel problem maintaining patterns.

Characteristic cognitions in different problems

CBT theories associate characteristic forms of cognition with particular kinds of problem. These characteristic patterns involve both the *content* of cognitions and the *process* of cognition.

Depression

As first described by Beck, a fundamental cognitive characteristic in depression is the *negative cognitive triad* (negatively biased views of *oneself*, of the *world in general* and of the *future*). The typical depressed view is that I am bad (useless, unlovable, incompetent, worthless, a failure, etc.), the world is bad (people are not nice to me, nothing good happens, life is just a series of trials), and the future is also bad (not only am I and the world bad, but it will always be like this and nothing I can do will make any difference).

Depressed people's thoughts are likely to contain not only characteristic *contents*, e.g. negative views of themselves or others, but also characteristic general biases in the *way* that they think, e.g. towards perceiving and remembering negative events more than positive ones, or tending to see anything that goes wrong as being their fault, or over-generalising from one small negative event to a broad negative conclusion.

Your best starting place for reading more about the cognitive theory of depression and its treatment is Beck et al.'s (1979) seminal text *Cognitive therapy of depression*. Later the CBT world embraced a revised theory and practice that was relevant to those suffering with *repeated* depressive episodes and mindfulness-based cognitive therapy (MBCT) was established (Teasdale, Segal & Williams, 1995). An excellent text updating the position of MBCT is Segal, Williams and Teasdale, 2018.

Anxiety

The general cognitive process here is a bias towards *the overestimation of threat* (i.e. perceiving a high risk of some unwanted outcome) and/or the *underestimation of ability to cope* (i.e. perceiving oneself as lacking necessary skills) (Beck et al., 1985). The exact nature of the threat, and therefore the content of cognitions, is different in different disorders. For example:

- in *panic*, there is a catastrophic misinterpretation of harmless anxiety symptoms as indicating some imminent disaster, e.g. dying or 'going mad';
- in *health anxiety*, there is a similar misinterpretation of harmless symptoms as indicating illness but on a longer timescale, e.g. 'I might have a disease that will kill me sometime in the future';

- in *social anxiety*, thoughts are about being negatively evaluated by others, e.g. 'They will think I am stupid (or boring, or peculiar …)';
- in *GAD*, thoughts are typically in the form of pervasive worries about uncertainty and threat.

My go-to book when working with anxiety disorders is *Cognitive-behavioural therapy for anxiety disorders* by Butler, Fennell and Hackmann (2008).

Anger

In anger, the thoughts are usually about other people's behaviour being *unfair*, breaking some implicit or explicit *rule*, or having hostile intent: 'They ought not to do that, it's not fair, they're trying to put me down.' Just as we saw with anxiety, rapid and extreme conclusions are drawn – thus illustrating the cognitive process and content that lead to anger. In both anxiety and anger this is fueled by adrenaline, reminding us of the interacting systems of psychological experiences.

The development of CBT for anger management has not been as extensive as the development for anxiety and depressive disorders and it has tended to focus on offenders and young persons. Nonetheless there is quite a body of research that indicates it is effective (see Henwood, Chou and Browne, 2015 for a meta-analysis). There are a few guides for working with the general public and a particularly useful one is a self-help text: *Overcoming anger and irritability* by Davies (2016). It is grounded in CBT and very readable for both therapist and patient.

SUMMARY

- CBT is a talking therapy that helps people change the way they feel by helping them change the way they think and behave.
- The initial (cognitive) focus is on automatic cognitions but therapists can work at 'deeper' levels, addressing the problems underlying assumptions and core beliefs. CBT works with images as well as words.
- It has a sound evidence base for many psychological disorders and is frequently endorsed by NICE.
- The approach tends to focus on the present – the here and now – and is underpinned by a relationship of empirical collaboration.

REFLECTION & ACTION

At the end of each chapter you will find a section that prompts you to reflect on what's been covered in the text. The format will be the same in each section and essentially you'll be asked 'What?', 'So what?' and 'Now what?'.

This is with good reason. Back in the 1930s John Dewy pioneered the notion of enhancing learning through reflection and this was further developed by others over the years. You are probably familiar with Lewin's (1946), Kolb's (1984) and Gibbs' (1988) learning cycles, all of which build on Dewy's ideas and incorporate the critical elements of thinking, analysing, planning and getting active. I am particularly fond of Borton's beautifully simple 1970s' take on this as it captures the essence of enhanced learning in an easy to remember heuristic.

So that's what you'll be invited to consider at the end of each chapter:

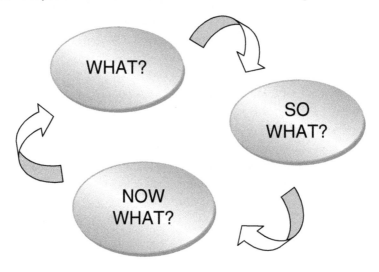

WHAT are you taking away from this chapter? What teaching points resonate with you?

....

....

....

....

....

....

....

....

....

....

SO WHAT? What significance do these points have – how do they relate to your previous learning or views? Do they challenge your former opinions? Have you gleaned new ideas for helping patients or indeed looking after your own needs?

....

....

....

....

....

....

....

....

....

....

NOW WHAT? This is all very well but how will you take this forward? What are you now going to do differently? Make a commitment with yourself to follow through on at least one of your new ideas.

....

....

....

....

....

....

....

....

....

FURTHER READING AND USEFUL WEBSITES

Beck, A.T., Rush, A.J., Shaw, B.F., & Emery, G. (1979). *Cognitive therapy of depression*. New York: Guilford Press.
The original CBT manual. Although now over forty years old, the book that started the cognitive revolution is still a classic, with a real feel for the clinical realities of working with depressed patients.

Butler, G., Fennell, M., & Hackmann, A. (2008). *Cognitive-behavioural therapy for anxiety disorders: mastering clinical challenges*. New York: Guilford Press.
Three wise and experienced clinician-researchers deliver what it says in their title, a comprehensive guide for a range of anxiety disorders. They show us how to build on individualised formulations, to work transdiagnostically and to integrate the art and science of CBT.

Greenberger, D., & Padesky, C. (2015). *Mind over mood* (2nd ed.). New York: Guilford Press.
A well–established and best-selling self-help book now in its second edition. It is designed to assist the general public, but it is also a clear and simple introduction to CBT that many new therapists find very useful, whether or not they plan to use it with patients.

Padesky, C., & Greenberger, G. (2020). *The clinician's guide to using Mind over Mood* (2nd ed.). New York: Guilford Press.
This is a very contemporary companion to using 'Mind over Mood' to its full advantage but, brimming with wisdom, it also stands alone as an excellent CBT guide.

Kennerley, H., Kirk, J., & Westbrook, D. (2017). *An introduction to cognitive behaviour therapy* (3rd ed.). London: Sage.
A popular introduction to CBT written by three CBT specialists. The book is comprehensive and readable and it is complemented by a companion website featuring over 40 videos illustrating CBT in practice.

Oxford Cognitive Therapy Centre (OCTC) www.octc.co.uk
OCTC was established over twenty-five years ago as a centre of excellence for CBT practice and its website provides direction for additional training and video access, CBT supervision and a number of useful downloadable documents.

The Centre for Outcomes Research & Effectiveness (CORE) www.ucl.ac.uk/clinical-psychology/CORE/CBT_Framework.htm
The CORE site contains more detailed descriptions of the CBT competences for anxiety and depression, and a self-assessment tool to allow clinicians to evaluate how well their own skills match the competences.

2

DEVELOPING A WORKING ALLIANCE

Now it's time to start thinking about putting CBT into action. You are entering an important relationship, sometimes a delicate relationship, and a good working alliance is integral to every session so that's where we begin.

YOUR WORKING ALLIANCE

Beck promotes the therapeutic relationship in CBT, using the terms 'working alliance' and 'therapeutic collaboration' (Beck et al., 1979: 45). This describes an active partnership of team-work and discovery where patient and therapist bring their own expertise and share responsibility for change. However, it is far from a business-like arrangement as it requires 'the same subtle therapeutic atmosphere that has been described explicitly in the context of psychodynamic psychotherapy ... relationship involves both the patient and the therapist and is based on trust, rapport and collaboration' (p. 50).

It has been long established that an effective therapist–patient relationship is important for treatment, with good evidence relating quality of relationship to therapeutic outcome (Orlinsky, Grawe & Parks, 1994). Its relevance is recognised by the BABCP as one of its accreditation criteria stipulates that a practitioner should 'Demonstrate knowledge and understanding of the therapeutic relationship and competence in the development, maintenance and ending of such relationships'. However, within CBT the therapeutic relationship is seen as necessary but not sufficient for a good treatment result, and in treatment trials there is typically a beneficial effect from CBT over and above that of being in a therapeutic relationship (Roth & Fonagy, 2005). Thus, we need to employ sound CBT strategies within a well-developed therapeutic relationship.

This begs the question: how is it done?

Building a collaborative therapeutic relationship

Fortunately, the guiding principles of CBT will help you build an authentic collaborative relationship as they encourage you to adopt an open-minded curiosity and respect about patients' beliefs, emotions and behaviours, without assuming that you know how they feel or think.

Another important aspect of building a good working relationship is demonstrating your respect for your patients' cognitive, emotional and life experiences and culture – it is crucial that you are sensitive to diversity, otherwise how can you devise a meaningful formulation that reflects your patients' inner worlds and experiences?

You should also attend to a person's readiness to change (Prochaska & DiClemente, 1986), pacing therapy accordingly, using motivational approaches (Miller & Rollnick, 2002) when necessary rather than 'active' CBT.

Consideration of these factors can ease the development of a good relationship from the outset. You can then work empathically and co-operatively, as a guide and mentor rather than as an instructor. Together you set your agenda, devise a shared formulation, establish agreed goals, and welcome mutual feedback. You are 'walking alongside' a patient, exploring new options for feeling and behaving; you ask questions and provide information that might open up previously unexplored areas; you reflect a genuine, concerned interest in that person's current perspectives or feelings.

This demands much active listening and enquiry, and the tone of the interaction is crucial: it shouldn't be accusatory ('You don't really mean you think that, do you?'), nor persuasive or haranguing ('Do you think it is possible that most people respond in this way and that you are not picking up the cues?'). We will sometimes need to press for detail and clarification, but there is a fine line between encouraging and haranguing or between suggesting and accusing, and we must strive to maintain sensitive, respectful enquiry.

Getting it just right every time can be challenging, particularly as we need to maintain a measure of skepticism about what our patients tell us. Remember that it is possible that cognitive biases are significantly distorting the picture a patient presents:

- 'I feel like this all of the time, there is no exception.'
- 'There is no-one to help me and there is nothing I can do.'
- 'Everyone is against me at work, just everyone.'

We need to build up an accurate picture of each patient's circumstances and abilities alongside a picture of their perception of reality at present. There is often a mismatch at the outset of therapy, and we explore this, looking for signs that there might be times of coping or support within a social network, but without giving the impression that we disbelieve our patient.

You also need to be flexible in your role within your working alliance, picking up on a patient's changing needs whilst still practising within the remit of your organisation and in the light of mutual resources. For example, you may need to carry out some of the therapeutic work outside the session because a home visit is called for or some in vivo practice is optimum;

you might need to bring in the patient's partner as an informant; you will certainly have to be flexible in shifting from Socratic guidance to offering information (see Chapters 7 and 8).

As well as providing information for reflection, you are a *practical scientist* offering models and hypotheses for consideration in relation to both current and future problems. Hypotheses are set up and tested, and new conclusions are drawn if appropriate. This type of interaction captures Beck's notion of 'collaborative empiricism' and hence is very relevant to building your working alliance. The adoption of an open-minded approach is essential throughout therapy, and the importance of looking for evidence that is at odds with your initial hypotheses is crucial. This is as true for the therapist's preliminary formulation as it is for the patient's initial beliefs. Evidence inconsistent with our ideas is the way to new perspectives!

The *collaborative* nature of the therapeutic relationship means that you relate in an adult-to-adult way. You are open about your ideas concerning a patient's problems and share your understandings of the formulation in a way that welcomes feedback on its relevance or accuracy; you may disclose information about yourself *if this is in your patient's interest*; and you are free to say 'I don't know' or 'Can I just think that over for a minute?'. Indeed, Beck tells us 'techniques … are intended to be applied in a tactful, therapeutic and human manner by a fallible person – the therapist' (Beck et al., 1979: 45–46).

The only exceptions to this openness are when it is clearly not in the patient's interest – tor example, you might choose not to disclose early in treatment your ideas about a possible final weight for a woman with anorexia nervosa lest you jeopardise her motivation to return to therapy and at least engage in weight stabilisation; you might not yet share your knowledge, gleaned from medical notes, of possible childhood abuse in case your patient is not ready to explore this – bringing it up might risk disengagement.

The therapeutic relationship can also be viewed as a useful laboratory for working on problems, providing an opportunity to acquire new skills and perspectives that can then be used outside the session. For example, a person might evaluate a 'hot' thought triggered in a therapy session or practise in-session relaxation or try out being assertive with the therapist, before applying this to real life.

Safran and Muran (1995) suggest that the therapist can provide new, constructive interpersonal experiences for a patient, with the patient and therapist stepping back together and examining what is currently going on between them. So, sessions might be used to review and modify unhelpful beliefs as they are played out with the therapist in the clinical setting before taking new perspectives into the world outside the therapy session.

Christina repeatedly 'lost' homework and then began to postpone sessions. Her therapist helped her share her fear of being criticised and rejected by him if the homework was not 'good enough.' He was able to give her the experience of being understood, not judged, and of being supported, not rejected. Christina could then update her interpersonal predictions: 'Some people will accept me for who I am and help me if I struggle.'

Alan predicted that others would not be there for him when he was in trouble. In a session where difficulties in the relationship seemed to be emerging, the therapist used her own feelings as the cue for a discussion, saying 'I am feeling rather uncertain of where to take things just now and I wonder why. It's my difficulty, I know, but could we explore this together?' The discussion revealed that Alan was uncertain whether or not the therapist could help him so he had been disinclined to engage in CBT, and he also predicted that she would 'sack him' if he didn't do well. They were then able to understand the tension in their relationship and went on to look at whether the therapist would be likely to withdraw if things became difficult, or whether she would want to find ways of persisting. This discussion was highly relevant to Alan's fears and led to the therapeutic relationship becoming a 'laboratory' for testing them.

Within this framework, the ways in which a patient responds to the therapist may be influenced by beliefs developed early in life (possibly modified by subsequent experience), as well as by the therapist's characteristics and behaviour. However, the therapeutic relationship is not construed in terms of 'transference', in the psychoanalytic sense that it is a representation of another relationship, but instead is considered as *a relationship in its own right*, with the potential for providing new evidence about the range of possibilities for relationships. For example, a new belief like 'People may stay with you even if difficulties emerge between you' may be strengthened. The extent to which a corrective interpersonal experience in therapy might colour other relationships should be considered empirically. If the issues are being openly discussed, it is easier to check out whether there is indeed generalisation to everyday life.

Establish your alliance as early on as possible – you don't want to risk losing your patient prematurely because you appear cold or unempathic – but this is not to say that the quality of the relationship remains fixed. It varies as treatment progresses, and it may be necessary to attend to breakdowns in the relationship in order for therapy to succeed. The quality of your therapeutic relationship should continue to be a focus of concern throughout the course of treatment.

Dealing with ruptures in your working alliance

Always be mindful of the quality of the interaction between you and your patient because ruptures in the working alliance do occur. Do not ignore these and hope that they will go away – it is wise to take early steps to intervene when difficulties arise.

These may be reflected in a patient's overt statements (e.g. 'I am not happy with this', 'You are judging me', 'I don't think you get it at all') and behaviours (e.g. not turning up for sessions, trying to give gifts) or through non-verbal cues (e.g. silences, avoiding eye contact, fidgeting). As a therapist you too might experience feelings or thoughts that could hinder therapy and these need to be addressed.

Safran and Segal (1990) describe an elegant way of addressing therapeutic ruptures that is generally Socratic (see Chapters 7 and 8) and certainly in keeping with the principles of CBT. In summary, their advice is as follows:

Observe the rupture. If you identify a recurring pattern first check that it is not the result of a simple misunderstanding that can be clarified. Never assume that it is a rift that is fundamental to your relationship. I recall things getting slightly, yet noticeably, tense with a patient and we addressed this only to discover that he was annoyed because I had started to arrive a minute or two late each session. This meant that we sometimes overran our original time and that stressed his wife who was waiting for him in a time-limited pick-up spot at the hospital. I explained that my delay was because a regular meeting had recently been moved to another building so it took me a few minutes longer to get to our session. Now that I appreciated that this stressed him, we could simply shift our start time: a successful practical solution that he hadn't realised was possible.

If the rupture seems to be related to your bond with your patient deal with this within your current therapeutic relationship and first consider what contribution you are making to any therapeutic impasse, rather than assume that the problem always resides within the patient. If it seems that the therapeutic relationship is being affected by your own issues or blind-spots, discuss this with your supervisor and take the opportunity to do some work yourself: for example, listen to recordings of your treatment sessions, keep a thought record and look for your own hot thoughts.

If it seems that the impasse is related to your patient's issues, then rather than viewing this as an indication of poor motivation or ambivalence or frank hostility, be open-minded and formulate the issue in the same way as any other problem. For example, consider what function behaviours might have, what idiosyncratic beliefs might fuel the impasse, what skills your patient might be lacking, etc. Do this without assuming that the problem is present across settings but if it is, then it may be necessary to consider the rupture as a characteristic pattern and you can use the therapeutic relationship to provide the patient with a corrective emotional experience (Safran & Muran, 1995).

Present the interpersonal issue as a dilemma for you as the therapist rather than using phrases that might imply that the patient is doing something that causes a problem.

Nina had suffered terrible developmental trauma and yet our sessions were lighthearted, and this seemed at odds with her past and current experiences. Rather than infer that she was avoiding exploring her grief and hurt I considered what I was struggling with so that we could use Socratic exploration that would not risk putting her on the defensive. I described my dilemma: 'I think that we could work better together, so is it okay if I run some ideas past you? I often feel that I don't really "get it". I listen to what you say, and I always find what you tell me really engaging. You are very clear and often entertaining, and I enjoy that. But I worry that while I'm enjoying the sessions I don't tune into your hurt and fears properly and that I could be doing you a disservice. I think I need help in appreciating just how difficult things are for you.' She acknowledged that she held back because of her own need to entertain and please people and her reservations about opening up and risking being overwhelmed by emotion. We could then formulate what was happening between us and develop some experiments to gently test her fears and predictions.

Later we looked at the possibility that the interpersonal patterns, uncovered in session, also played out in her life in general and she was able to see that, yes, with some people she behaved in the same way and that the work that we had done in the session might generalise to 'real life'.

Thus, we were able to identify the impasse and resolve a way through that was true to the collaborative spirit of CBT.

Boundary issues

At risk of stating the obvious, the relationship between therapist and patient is different from other social relationships, and boundary issues need careful and serious consideration in CBT, just as they do in other approaches. The main governing principles, common to all therapeutic encounters are:

- the patient's needs have primacy;
- gratification of the therapist's needs (beyond professional satisfaction and safety) is not acceptable.

The therapist must also feel safe. This can be achieved by ensuring that there are sensible policies about the kinds of referral accepted, that risk is properly assessed, and the physical location and arrangement of the clinic/sessions takes account of safety.

The extensive self-disclosure and neediness of the patient coupled with the power attributed to therapists means that even in the relatively collaborative CBT setting the therapeutic relationship is not equal. Throughout, it is the responsibility of the therapist, not the patient, to maintain boundaries, so you must seek sufficient supervision and support if you are concerned about boundary issues.

From time to time it may be beneficial to make home visits or accompany patients in everyday situations, for example in order to do an in-vivo experiment (see Chapter 8) or to observe a patient whose obsessional rituals prevent them from starting the day. Never undertake this lightly. Consider necessary safeguards to reduce the possibility of misinterpretations of your behaviour: for example, take along an assistant or include a relative in the session.

Therapist experiences may even be disclosed, *if this is appropriate* to the on-going task. For example:

Colin had fears about sweating heavily, particularly in places with bright lights. The therapist arranged a couple of treatment sessions in a bright café where she wet her face, back, and armpits to look as though she was sweating heavily. Colin sat nearby, observing the responses of the waiter and other people. Colin then asked the therapist what thoughts were going through her mind, and how she felt in the situation.

It is helpful to make the aims of such sessions very explicit, by spending time agreeing what predictions are being tested, how the experiment will be conducted, and so on. This makes good technical sense and also sets boundaries, making it clear that this is a treatment session with a specific purpose, and not a social event. This can be difficult for some patients to accept, especially if the therapist contact is the only social event of the week.

Finally, the collaborative style of CBT can sometimes be compromised if the therapist is involved in a compulsory admission to an institution. The repercussions can be minimised if (i) you have already discussed this possibility and how it would be approached, or (ii) you discuss at the time and/or after the crisis what it means to your patient. In this way you can continue to be as open as possible while offering an empathic ear, clarifying misperceptions and, if possible, moving towards problem-solving and planning.

It was very clear that Mel was at risk of attempting suicide if she went home alone after the session. Her therapist reminded her that they had discussed that, at times like these, the therapist would have to involve the psychiatric team. Mel was not happy to hear this, but she was not surprised by her therapist's position. Her therapist ran through the next steps with Mel: she explained that she would make a phone call to the duty doctor – one that Mel could listen to – and that she would walk with Mel to the hospital reception where the psychiatrist would assess her. She offered to stay with Mel until the doctor arrived and also explained that if Mel were admitted, she would visit her on the ward to continue the sessions, if that's what Mel wanted. She then asked Mel what she thought of this arrangement. Mel was still unhappy, but she was relieved that her therapist was not angry and was not going to discharge her. She was also reassured that her therapist was open and honest.

SUMMARY

- Cognitive therapy invests in an open, collaborative and empathic therapeutic relationship.
- We work within this therapeutic alliance to engender realistic hope, encourage motivation and manage ruptures.
- Ruptures are addressed using open and Socratic methods in keeping with the general approach of CBT.
- We also work within a boundaried relationship where responsibility for ethical practice rests with the therapist.

REFLECTION & ACTION

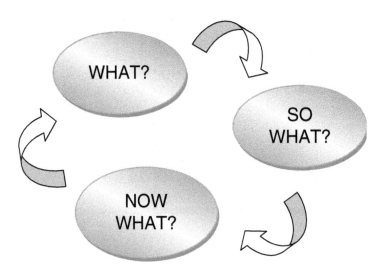

WHAT are you taking away from this chapter? What teaching points resonate with you?

....
....
....
....
....
....
....
....
....
....

SO WHAT? What significance do these points have – how do they relate to your previous learning or views? Do they challenge your former opinions? Have you gleaned new ideas for helping patients or indeed looking after your own needs?

....

....

....

....

....

....

....

....

....

....

NOW WHAT? This is all very well but how will you take this forward? What are you now going to do differently? Make a commitment with yourself to follow through on at least one of your new ideas.

....

....

....

....

....

....

....

....

....

....

3

STRUCTURING YOUR CBT SESSION

CBT is relatively brief and careful structuring helps us get the most from each session. Each session is shaped by an agenda which, along with capsule summaries, helps us keep on track. The entire arc of therapy is guided by well-specified goals and sessions are linked by relevant, active assignments.

AGENDA-SETTING

This is not a superficial opening gambit; it is important on many levels and therefore we need to look at it closely. Agenda-setting contributes to using time effectively by:

- providing an overt framework for the session (thus promoting the structure);
- prioritising the issues to be addressed in a session (thus maintaining focus).

Agendas usually comprise:

- *a brief review of events or time between sessions* – this would include a mood update, reflections on the previous session (what was helpful and what could have improved the session) and there would be an emphasis on reviewing assignments: issues raised here might be carried over to the session's main topics;
- *main topics for discussion* – these may include symptoms and/or crises or might focus on working on particular CBT skills, such as learning how to identify ATs, or the role of safety-seeking behaviours in the maintenance of problems: it is often necessary to *prioritise* items as only a few can be covered in the session;

- *homework/assignment* – this should arise from the main topics as they are discussed, so it may already have been negotiated well before the end of the session: however, it is worth allowing time to ensure that assignments have been set up properly;
- *feedback on the experience of the session* – you need to make sure you have left time on the agenda to ask for feedback on what was helpful about the session and what could have made it even better: ensure that your patient reflects on the learning points and can see how to take these forward.

But there is more to the agenda: asking a patient what they wish to add is collaborative, thereby developing the working alliance and engaging the patient as an active participant. It is also an exercise promoting problem-solving: we ask patients to clarify key issues, to be specific and to prioritise – all necessary skills for learning how to problem-solve. Finally, it is an exercise in reflective learning because it opens with a review, reflection or debriefing of assignments, and ends with a summing-up of learning points and clarifying plans for homework.

A strong rationale for agenda-setting should be presented at the outset of treatment. For example:

'CBT is a time limited therapy so it's important that we get the most out of the time we have. That's why we'll always start with an agenda. This means that items that are relevant to you and to me get a slot and that we use the session as efficiently as we can. I usually have ideas about what I would like to include, but you will want to discuss things that have happened in the week, or thoughts that have occurred to you, and so on. So it would be helpful if you could take a few minutes before each session just thinking over what you would like to include. We can then agree an agenda between us. Does that sound sensible? Would you be willing to have a go at that?'

Ask what your patient wants to cover, and then suggest your relevant items. Make each item specific so that you both know what to focus on and you can review your progress in addressing that issue – vague notions of what to do in the session lend themselves neither to focus nor review. You also need to ensure that the item is relevant to your patient's problem. For example, someone might bring along a recent issue of becoming overwhelmed when completing benefits forms. Consider if this is relevant to their main problem. Maybe it is because being overwhelmed is a recurring theme and their depression is exacerbated by their not being able to think things through clearly and subsequent self-criticism. However, the benefits forms might reflect a more practical stressor and not be directly relevant to the depression. Then, a more effective solution would be to consult a friend or the mental health team's social worker.

The process of screening and refining items for the agenda may take a few minutes at the start of each session – this is time well spent but it means there is limited time for the major topics for the day. Therefore, usually no more than two or three main topics can be included. These items need to be prioritised according to:

- risk to patient or others;
- urgency, e.g. possible job loss, imminent exams;
- level of distress;
- centrality to the formulation;
- potential for change;
- relevance to a skill that needs to be learned;
- whether the problem could be tackled with someone else outside therapy.

If possible, you might want to consider including more complex problems on the agenda later in therapy when your patient has the skills to deal with them effectively. However, balance this against the advantage of dealing with issues that are seen as important by the patient or that have a genuine urgency.

The final item on an agenda is usually 'feedback'. This is where patient and therapist can comment on what they have learnt from the session and what they might build on. You need to make sure that there is sufficient time to do this properly and you might introduce the idea using statements such as the following:

'We want to make sure that these sessions suit you, so it would be helpful to have your views on how things were today: what has gone well and perhaps how things might have gone even better. I appreciate that it may be difficult at first to tell me if things have been disappointing, or if I have said something that has upset you, but it is really helpful to tell me whether things are okay or not … What would you say are the take-home messages from today? … Is there anything else that has been helpful, that we should build on? … Can you think how things might have been even better? … Is there anything I have said that is going to play on your mind, or has been unhelpful? … Any other comments on today?

What I would like to feedback to you is that I'm impressed by the way that you are open-minded and consider different options – that will stand you in good stead in CBT because we explore different perspectives and possibilities and we can really build on the skill that you already have. Also, I am really heartened by the way that you have been open to exploring difficult issues. This will help us properly understand your problems. Between now and when we next meet, you might want to think about ways in which I can make it easier or more comfortable for you to look at difficult issues.'

Once the agenda items are prioritised and agreed, consider roughly how much time each issue needs. Timing is not set in stone as we have to be responsive to unforeseen needs, but it is good to have a 'ballpark' idea of time allocation to guide you through the session. Otherwise it is all too easy to run out of time. A tip from my colleague Dr Gillian Butler is to write the agenda on your whiteboard so that it is visible and you are reminded of your plan for the session. Follow your agenda and be explicit about deviations from it. For example, if your patient moves to a different topic don't just go along with it assuming that they would choose to prioritise the new topic. Instead, flag it and discuss it, by saying something like:

'I notice that you've shifted to talking about your eating patterns, which makes me think this might be an important issue. Would you like us to review our agenda and spend some of our time thinking about this, or would you rather that we focus instead on flashbacks, as we agreed at the beginning of the session? We can be flexible.'

This allows your patient to review the relevance of the digression and make a choice. Digressions might not be relevant to the presenting problem and issues shouldn't be taken up just because they are of interest. In the above example, the patient might have difficulty controlling her weight but this could be irrelevant to her PTSD, in which case she might seek help elsewhere or simply put the topic on hold while she focuses on her trauma work. On the other hand, she could be binge-eating to combat flashbacks, thus the eating behaviour is intrinsic to her PTSD and it would be appropriate to give it floor space and formulate this. It goes without saying that if the discussion brings up a topic related to risk, you will review your agenda, and prioritise risk issues over other items.

It is common to encounter some difficulties setting and sticking to an agenda, but you can minimise the likelihood of problems by ensuring:

- It is specific – clarify precisely what your patient needs to address and don't waste time.
- It is realistic – avoid too many items.
- It has genuine input from your patient.

Also:

- Tackle topics *after* you have set the agenda – avoid picking up items as soon as they are mentioned and only introduce new items following an agenda review.

Finish one item, summarise and consider action points before moving on to the next item.

CAPSULE SUMMARIES

Capsule summaries are brief summaries capturing where you are in the session, reviewing the main points of the discussion. These are invaluable in keeping you on track. Aim to summarise every five to 10 minutes and certainly at the closure of a topic – this will help you keep to your agenda and provide a useful break between topics.

Initially as the therapist we offer the summary but later we might ask patients to do this, as it helps them learn the skill of taking stock. To check out that your summary is valid, you could ask questions such as:

'You seem to be saying …
Do I have that right?
Have I missed anything?'

But remember that you can also elicit summaries from patients:

'Could you put in your own words what you see as the main points of our discussion and how we can take things forward?'

GOAL-SETTING

Another aspect of CBT that helps maintain its efficiency as a time-limited therapy is working towards mutually agreed and clearly specified goals. Goal-setting implies the possibility of progress, which engenders hope and reduces helplessness in the face of what may seem insurmountable problems. It also raises the prospect of treatment ending, and helps you openly negotiate discharge.

This is not a task to take lightly, care must be taken to ensure that the goals are meaningful and that they are clearly defined.

Meaningful goals

A first step in ensuring that goals are meaningful is to derive them jointly. By doing this they will have relevance for the patient – and the collaborative nature of CBT will be emphasised as a helpful by-product.

Goals should also reflect your shared formulation. For example, if someone is depressed and you identify maintaining cycles of inactivity and rumination, your targets should embrace this.

Sometimes, patients express goals such as 'to lose weight', 'to get on better with my part-ner': before you both accept these as goals, check that they are relevant to therapy, that they are indicated by the formulation, that they are *meaningful*. It's possible that low mood is genu-inely exacerbated by weight gain driven by comfort-eating, so this would then be an appro-priate issue to target. On the other hand, some expressions are simply 'wishes' that might be desirable for the patient but not relevant to therapy. So, if a patient is overweight but their eating patterns and weight do not actively contribute to the maintenance of depression, then weight loss could be tackled elsewhere.

Clearly defined goals

To help your patient develop their goals, begin with general questions:

'Let's imagine that therapy has been successful – what would be different? What changes would you see?'

'At the end of treatment, what would you like to be different?'

The so-called 'miracle question' is sometimes a good way of getting at goals:

'Imagine a miracle happens, all your problems disappear while you sleep. When you get up the next morning and go through your day, how will you come to realise the miracle has happened? What would you notice was different about you or about other people? What would you do differently? What will have changed? What would *others* see that would tell them the miracle had happened?'

If you read about negotiating goals in therapy, you will usually find a recommendation that goals be 'SMART'. Confusingly, different sources use this acronym differently, but a typical suggestion is that goals should be:

- **S**pecific
- **M**easurable
- **A**chievable
- **R**ealistic
- and have a realistic **T**imeframe (i.e. a date for completion).

At this point, I have to own up to using simpler standards. I find **S**pecific, **A**chievable and **M**easurable (SAM) criteria sufficient to ensure the development and evaluation of goals. A colleague adds a second 'M' for Meaningful, making the acronym 'SAMM'. As far as I know there is no CBT research that tells us if 'SMART' is better than 'SAM' or 'SAMM' so it's up to you really. But here are the reasons for at least aiming for 'SAM'.

Setting out goals in *specific* detail can help a person feel more in control, because a global problem reduced to its component parts may seem more manageable. So, once you have some general ideas, refine them.

For example, if your patient has the goal of 'socialising more', we need to know the following:

- With whom?
- When?
- Where?
- For how long?
- How often?

This precision helps plan specific steps in achieving the goal and makes progress transparent and measurable. An imprecise notion of when and where can lead to fuzzy planning and difficulty in recognising achievements.

Heidi was preoccupied by health worries, particularly concerning breast cancer. Her therapist asked how she might know that treatment had been successful. She replied:

> I would stop checking myself for lumps … I wouldn't be thinking about cancer all the time and boring the family. The main thing is I wouldn't get panicky every time cancer was mentioned.

Heidi's response reveals a common problem: she described how she would like *not* to be, rather than how she would like to *be*. My former boss called this the 'dead man's solution', meaning the goals could be achieved by a dead man – no more panicky feelings, no more checking lumps, no more talking to relatives about cancer. Ask how your patients want to be or what they want to achieve, rather than what they want to avoid.

The 'miracle question' helped Heidi develop goals that were about achievements:

1. Carry out a full breast check (procedure agreed upon by Heidi and therapist) on a monthly basis.

2. Discuss topics other than cancer symptoms (e.g. local news, update on how work was going) with my husband 100% of the time.
3. Visit relatives (alone or with a companion) in the local hospital.
4. Respond calmly if I think I have symptoms – relax (achieving 5/10 or lower on a 10-point scale).

These are four *specific* goals: Heidi and the therapist are quite clear about what indicates a success.

Goals can be daunting – if they were easily attained our patients wouldn't need help – so we need to maintain hope and motivation. To make the challenge less off-putting and create a plan that enabled progress to be measured, Heidi was asked to consider the realistic steps she could take to achieve each goal. She then devised a hierarchy of steps (sometimes called 'graded tasks') beginning with what she could do right now (at a push):

Possible now: Daily full breast checks on rising and before going to bed. Mini-checks at odd times during the day.

Step 1: Daily full breast checks on rising and before going to bed only.

Step 2: Daily full breast checks on going to bed only.

Step 3: Full breast checks every other day on going to bed.

Step 4: Full breast checks Monday and Thursday only (Heidi chooses timing from now on).

Step 5: Full breast checks once per week.

Step 6: Full breast checks once per fortnight.

Goal: Monthly full breast checks.

Progress can be measured by changes in her behaviour. If a simple self-rating were included at each step – say a 1–10 anxiety scale or a thought log – then this would make her progress measures more informative.

This series of tasks is not immutable. With each step Heidi's confidence and perspectives would be reviewed and the steps might be refined and changed. Breaking down a goal like this can impart hope and improve motivation. It can transform the seemingly impossible to the believably achievable.

Part of your role is to make sure that goals are achievable (i.e. *realistic*). People sometimes have unrealistic goals: a socially anxious person wanting to find a life partner by the end of therapy, for example. Sometimes goals are too limited, such as someone with obsessional disorder wanting to reduce their hand-washing to four hours a day. Occasionally it may be difficult for patient and therapist to agree on goals. Consider the person with anorexia nervosa who wants help to lose weight; or someone with OCD wanting help to make their rituals more thorough. Delicate negotiation is required, but this process allows therapists and patients to be explicit about what can and cannot be achieved through therapy.

Colin had obsessional concerns about completing forms and the goal of 'Being absolutely certain I have filled in all forms correctly.'

> Therapist: You'd like to be *absolutely* certain that you've made no errors, and at present that means that you check at least a dozen times. Can you put yourself in the shoes of someone who no longer has OCD – what might your goal be?
>
> Colin: I suppose I'd aim not to check at all. Just fill in the form.
>
> Th: Does that sound a reasonable goal? To fill in forms without checking them.
>
> C: No – I think everyone probably checks things like that once.
>
> Th: Okay. So what would be a reasonable goal?
>
> C: Perhaps checking once (really important forms twice), without going over it in my head or anything.
>
> Th: Sounds reasonable – and what about feeling 'absolutely certain' that you've made no errors? Is that possible?
>
> C: I don't think so. I want to be certain but if I'm only going to check once then I'll probably have to accept not feeling 'absolutely certain'. To be honest even when I check and check I never feel that.

His goal for successful treatment was now less rigorous but more realistic.

Achievable goals involve change within a person's control: in particular, changing things about themself rather than other people. While it may be reasonable to have job-seeking as a goal, being offered a job is determined by someone else, and therefore may not be achievable. It is also worth considering whether the person has the resources – finance, skills, persistence, time, social support – to achieve the goals. Someone with limited income might not be able to adopt a BE that involves several train journeys, as this is expensive; a single parent without childcare will not be able to carry out multiple solo experiments.

When considering the timeframe, remember that you would not necessarily expect to see someone achieve all their goals before discharge. The important thing is that they have the skills to attain goals and this might be in their own time. Heidi was discharged when she had only reached Step 4 of her initial hierarchy, but she was clearly capable of making systematic behavioural changes and at follow-up she had taken herself to the final level of only checking monthly. She had not addressed all her goals in therapy as there had been no opportunity to visit relatives in hospital, but her therapist had prompted her to generalise from her experience of tackling other goals and was confident that Heidi knew the general strategy for goal attainment.

The choice of goal(s) to take first is determined by factors similar to those for prioritising topics in a session. It is usually helpful to opt for a goal where rapid change is possible, as this increases hope, engagement and motivation. Other determining factors include risk, urgency, importance or level of distress. Sometimes a goal logically needs to be approached before others can be tackled (for example, a person would need to be able to travel to an interview before they could interview for a post, and so would need to tackle anxiety about travelling before addressing anxiety about interviews).

As steps towards a goal are achieved and when the goal itself is reached, remember this was a means to an end – the result being a shift in cognition and affect. So always check in:

'What does doing X mean to you – and knowing that how do you feel?'

Also encourage ongoing progress by asking: 'What will you do differently as a result?'

For the therapist, another consideration is the ethical acceptability of the goal. For example, someone might want to reduce their distress when experiencing violent images about harming others, rather than address the images themselves. This person would be encouraged to consider the personal meaning of the images and the consequences of maintaining them. In this case the relevant intervention might be anger management.

HOMEWORK OR ASSIGNMENTS

Most problems occur outside the clinic and patients best learn through direct experience where it matters. So, it is not surprising that people who complete between-session assignments show greater improvement than those who do not (Kazantzis, Deane & Ronan, 2002; Schmidt & Woolaway-Bickel, 2000). This is probably partly because they have more opportunity to apply what they have learnt to everyday life and they consolidate their learning and confidence.

CBT views the patient as an apprentice learning to become their own therapist. Thus, assignments are central to CBT and time must be allocated to devising them, usually five or 10 minutes during or at the end of a session. Homework will often follow on directly from major topics on the agenda and will be evolved mid-session as part of that discussion. For example, if the topic concerned negative cognitions triggering anxious feelings, an obvious between-session task might be monitoring triggers and thoughts associated with anxiety; a discussion about the role of food cravings in someone with binge-eating disorder, might lead to homework involving monitoring urges to binge, or experimenting with distraction to see what effect this has on cravings.

The range of possible assignments is boundless, but they must be relevant to progressing towards treatment goals. Meaningful tasks can include reading pertinent material; listening to treatment recordings; self-monitoring feelings, thoughts or behaviours; carrying out experiments; practising new skills such as using thought records or being assertive; activity scheduling. Whatever you opt for, assignments must make sense to the patient, and they should be useful either for the subsequent treatment session, or for the achievement of a particular goal. For example, the results from a behavioural experiment may feed directly into the next session, where those results could flesh out the formulation, and then lead on to the next assignment.

If homework has been completed, or nearly completed, then it should be reviewed in detail. For example, if your patient has read a chapter of a book, what was helpful? What rang bells for them? Were there any sections that were difficult to understand? If they have completed an activity schedule, what was the pattern of pleasure, purposefulness and achievements? What did they learn? How can this be taken forward?

Sometimes homework is not done. Anticipate this. Assignments can be neglected for a number of reasons:

- Practical explanations: workload unexpectedly increasing; lack of money to carry out a task in a social situation, for example.
- Misunderstanding.
- Homework forgotten: perhaps because it was not discussed in sufficient detail, or not written down.
- Task too difficult.

Always explore why not completing an assignment is understandable – so much can be learnt from this. In fact, welcome it in the early days as it often gives us the chance to better understand a person's situation and fears. Difficult tasks can be modified for a subsequent assignment, or perhaps carried out with assistance from you or someone else.

If underlying beliefs have interfered with the completion of the task then tackle this pragmatically, at least initially, rather than attempting premature belief change. For example, if it seems that your patient has beliefs about control or autonomy that have been activated by a particular assignment, then the task could be modified to give them more control:

Robin did not do homework on two consecutive weeks. When this was reviewed, he raised concerns about the relevance of the tasks, although he had not mentioned this when the homework was agreed. The therapist wondered whether autonomy might be an issue for him, but did not raise it at this early stage in therapy, particularly as it did not seem to be related to the problems Robin had initially presented. Instead, it was agreed that Robin would play a bigger role in setting up homework. This meant that often tasks were weightier than the therapist would have suggested, but by and large were completed.

Nonetheless, you do need to consider that underlying beliefs do sometimes interfere with completing assignments. For instance, someone with perfectionist beliefs may find activity scheduling difficult to complete because they might think that none of their activities were challenging enough to include, or someone with low self-esteem may find it difficult to do a task where the outcome could be construed as falling short of the therapist's 'wishes'.

The following 'top-tips' can increase the likelihood that homework is attempted and is useful:

- Let homework *follow logically* from what happened in session and devise it *during* the session if it fits well there: you don't have to wait until the end of the session to discuss assignments.
- Make assignments relevant. Check this out with questions such as 'Does this make sense?', 'Can you summarise for me how you think this would be helpful?'
- People have lives outside of therapy so be *realistic* in your planning.
- Plan homework *in detail*, spelling out what is to be done, when, where, with whom, etc. Identify pitfalls and difficulties by asking carefully what could prevent the task being carried out.
- Ensure that homework *cannot be 'failed'*; see it as a source of helpful information, whatever the outcome. For example, if someone is attempting to reduce avoidance of particular situations, set up homework so that they can collect useful information about anxious thoughts and feelings even if they cannot reduce the avoidance.
- Provide *relevant resources*, such as record forms or reading material, at least early in therapy.

- The agreed assignments should be *noted down* by both of you because details get forgotten. Although it may be quicker for you to write it down *for* your patient, it is helpful to establish their active role in therapy.
- *Homework review* should always be on the agenda of the subsequent session, partly because it should have been designed to be relevant for the session, but also because none of us is likely to persist with assignments that are never followed up.

The key message is that it is important to establish from the outset that homework is an integral part of therapy, and that it is difficult to proceed without the information and feedback that it provides. This is particularly true when the amount of treatment is limited by resource constraints. Well-devised homework can mean that very limited treatment time can result in enormous changes as much of the work is done outside sessions.

SUMMARY

CBT is a time-limited therapy so we structure sessions and the course of therapy to maximise opportunities by adopting the following:

- Setting an agenda to keep the session relevant and focused.
- Using capsule summaries to review and keep us on track.
- Defining therapy goals to guide us over the course of treatment.
- Agreeing between-session assignments to maintain momentum and maximise outcome.

REFLECTION & ACTION

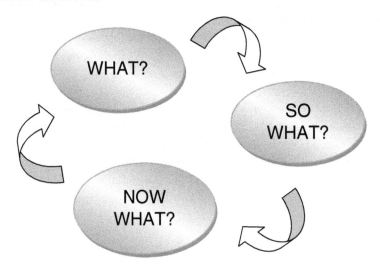

WHAT are you taking away from this chapter? What teaching points resonate with you?

....

....

....

....

....

....

....

....

....

....

SO WHAT? What significance do these points have – how do they relate to your previous learning or views? Do they challenge your former opinions? Have you gleaned new ideas for helping patients or indeed looking after your own needs?

....

....

....

....

....

....

....

....

....

....

NOW WHAT? How will you now address structuring your session? What are you now going to do differently? Make a commitment with yourself to follow through on at least one of your new ideas.

....

....

....

....

....

....

....

....

....

....

4

STRUCTURING A COURSE OF CBT

Just as a CBT session is structured, the entire course of treatment follows a considered arc with recognisable stages. Sometimes the arc is relatively short – for most straightforward problems, a course of therapy typically takes six to 15 hour-long sessions. However, there are no hard and fast rules about the length or the number of sessions. This is kept under review and informed by the patient's current formulation and our knowledge of best practice.

The UK National Institute for Health and Clinical Excellence (NICE) reviews research, synthesises guidelines for best practice, and provides advice concerning length of treatment. NICE recommendations should always be considered and balanced with patient needs. The ideal CBT is adaptable.

The ideal CBT is also always responsive to need. Sessions may be longer than an hour if they include in vivo behavioural experiments, shorter towards the end of treatment; the number of sessions may be extended if problems are more complex or the patient goes into crisis, shortened if the problem is highly amenable to treatment; therapy might be suspended temporarily to accommodate a patient's life events, such as giving birth, taking a lengthy holiday, starting a new job.

Sessions are usually weekly to begin with, and gradually less frequent as treatment progresses, perhaps with a couple of follow-up sessions. Of course, the amount and type of intervention offered is sometimes directed by others, e.g. where insurance companies dictate the level of intervention or the situation where a person can only afford a limited amount of therapy. Thus, you need to use limited time wisely.

The initial sessions will usually focus on assessing problem(s), deriving a shared formulation, developing your working relationship, educating your patient about CBT and their expected role. The final couple of sessions are concerned with drawing up a post-discharge blueprint, and the sessions in-between involve the active work on target problems, reviewing the formulation and goals and learning how to manage relapses.

EARLY STAGES

The crucial first step in therapy is engagement. Your knowledge of establishing a therapeutic alliance is invaluable at this stage, and coupling this with psychoeducation gives your patient a sound rationale for engaging in therapy as well as the sense of a safe foundation. It is helpful to *understand* reluctance to engage, rather than assuming 'poor motivation'. Try to analyse the problem in terms of thoughts, feelings and behaviours, so that you can generate ideas about managing the problem.

Below are some common obstacles to engagement:

- *Inaccurate expectations about treatment.* It is crucial to give clear information about CBT and a clear indication of what engaging in therapy involves.
- *Lack of understanding or acceptance of the formulation.* Invest time clarifying the formulation, gathering feedback, listening to concerns, and trying to take account of them. If you and your patient have not agreed on a formulation or the cognitive-behavioural approach by around session 4 or 5 you might need to consider that CBT is not the right therapy for this person, at least not at the moment, and that other forms of therapy are worth considering.
- *Hopelessness.* Hopelessness is common in depressed people, but it may affect those with a history of unsuccessful psychological treatments. Approach this using standard CBT techniques, including identifying and evaluating negative automatic thoughts and devising experiments focused on hopelessness.
- *Ambivalence about change.* Prochaska and DiClemente (1986) defined a spectrum of stages in a person's preparedness to change: not everyone is at the optimum stage of readiness when they enter therapy. As motivation tends to increase with more successful experiences, try to set up success experiences early on and keep motivation under review, as it can change as therapy proceeds.

Cost and benefits of CBT

Part of our work is uncovering obstacles to engagement and helping our patients feel that CBT is worth a try. Remember that therapy might have costs for the patient: emotional strain, investing time and possibly money, and implications for other changes in a person's life, changes that can seem risky. We often ask patients to make changes that require courage, and they are only likely to do that if they see possible benefits outweighing probable costs.

Cost–benefit matrices can be illuminating for reluctant or ambivalent patients. These go beyond a simple listing of immediate pros and cons by prompting consideration of both the short- and long-term implications:

Freya, who had a severe vomit phobia, was finding it difficult to give up safety-seeking behaviours (SSBs) even though she understood the rationale for doing so. Her cost–benefit analysis for dropping the behaviours is shown in Figure 4.1.

Freya could now look beyond her short-term fears and consider the long-term benefits. Even at a glance she could see that the benefits outweighed the costs but she could also see that it was no wonder that she hung on to her SSBs as they were effective in short-term. This new perspective enabled her to dare to drop her safety-seeking behaviours.

Short-term costs	Short-term benefits
Panicky at the time Anxious all day Nauseous Might be sick Worry about the mess	Feel I was doing something for the problem Feel less weak and out of control
Long-term costs	**Long-term benefits**
Might have to do harder and harder things No excuse to avoid the places I don't want to visit!	Gain confidence in my ability to cope with problems Better chance of overcoming my phobia, and then I could: go out freely; travel more widely, go abroad; eat more foods; be calm; be comfortable at formal events; use restaurants; feel more adult; relax about cleanliness in the home

Figure 4.1   Cost–benefit matrix: the consequences of giving up safety-seeking behaviours

Although this type of analysis will often encourage moving forward, you should consider that occasionally patients decide that, on balance, the costs of therapy outweigh the benefits for them right now. In such instances, be prepared to carry out more motivational work but also to recognise when CBT is not a compelling intervention for your patient and other interventions (or none at all) might be more appropriate.

Cognitions in the early stages

Most patients readily engage with the cognitive aspect of CBT, but on occasion there are problems.

Many will be able to identify key cognitions, even in the early stages of therapy, but sometimes you will hear patients say 'I don't have any thoughts.' Often this is simply a skills deficit – this person just isn't used to targeting cognitions. Many patients will be able to develop this ability, but it might require a preparation period. If so, they could begin by identifying what situations mean in a general sense, even if specific cognitions aren't readily accessible at first. As cognitions are central to CBT, it is important to deal with this early on and Chapter 7 discusses more ways of helping patients pinpoint mental events.

Another potential stumbling block is that some patients' understanding of the role of cognitions is different from a CBT view. For example, some patients with obsessional worries may explain their intrusions in terms of a religious framework or those with somatic symptoms may often construe symptoms purely in terms of physical illness. Be curious – try to find a way of working with this, as an experiment, without appearing to attack the patient's view. Negotiate trying an alternative understanding (based on a CBT formulation) as an experiment to see whether it works any better than the religious understanding or the physical illness formulation. Chapter 5 explores personalised formulations.

Sometimes patients will have differing beliefs about the roles and responsibilities of therapists (e.g. 'It's your job to cure me'). You could then devise assignments to draw attention to the important contribution that the patient can make to therapy. A useful metaphor is that of a road map – the therapist's knowledge can put you on the right page of the map, but you need the detailed information that only the patient has to direct you along the right roads. You then need to set up experiments which demonstrate that this collaborative approach can be helpful.

Relapse management

You might wonder why *relapse management* is introduced in the early stages of therapy and why it's not called *relapse prevention*. The term 'management' is used because aiming for 'prevention' is often unrealistic. In general, people will have setbacks and that they need to learn the necessary skills to deal with them – and the earlier a skill is introduced the more it can be refined. Relapse management is revisited in Chapter 9, so it is simply flagged up here.

Review points

CBT is time-limited and focused so requires regular reviews throughout treatment. This keeps CBT focused and helps establish whether progress is sufficient to warrant continuing, or whether changes in the approach are required. Reviews should relate to goals and it is helpful if intermediate targets have been identified, as well as end-point goals. Other measures, such as questionnaires or self-monitoring indices, are also relevant for taking stock at reviews.

At the outset, agree to review progress after a few sessions so you can assess whether CBT is likely to be helpful. Set this up so that it is clear that CBT is being reviewed for its suitability for the patient, that this is not just about the patient's application to CBT. Although a decision to discontinue CBT may be dispiriting, it is easier to deal with this at an early stage rather than after many sessions have resulted in little change. After this initial review, repeat the re-evaluation every five or so sessions depending on the length of the intervention.

Your initial formulation is tentative, so it is important to review and revise it regularly to incorporate new information that becomes available as therapy progresses. This may come from assignments, in-session behavioural experiments and so on. Although the basic outline of the formulation may not change, the details of maintaining cycles are often fleshed out and refined during treatment, with implications for what interventions are likely to be helpful.

Gerard, who had agoraphobia, was unclear about the content of his catastrophic thinking because he had avoided situations that triggered such thoughts. Once he had learnt to 'catch' ATs it became evident that he had thoughts about not being helped by other people. These thoughts could now be detailed in the formulation, and experiments set up to test them.

It is especially important to review progress if little change is being made, or if an impasse has been reached. This may be for many reasons, but it could mean that the formulation is not helpful or has significant omissions (another good reason for reviewing your shared conceptualisation). It is also worth looking at the therapeutic relationship to see whether there are problems interfering with the application of the formulation (see Chapter 2). Such problems may include your own blind spots or sensitivities, which could be discussed with your supervisor. If no way forward can be found, you may conclude that treatment simply isn't helpful at this point and you can begin to explore alternative options with your patient.

LATER STAGES

As treatment progresses, the emphasis is on intervention rather than assessment, but the results of any intervention should always be related back to the initial formulation to see whether it needs modifying. By now your patient should be increasingly independent in determining what items will go onto the agenda, what homework is taken away etc., and as more CBT skills are learnt then patients take the lead in, for example, evaluating negative thoughts and in devising behavioural experiments to test out new perspectives and possibilities.

You will probably focus on the details of automatic thoughts, feelings and behaviour in current situations in your sessions, but as treatment progresses you may begin to identify and evaluate unhelpful assumptions or core beliefs, particularly if you think that your patient may be at risk of relapse if these kinds of cognitions are not modified. It is, however, not always necessary to address underlying beliefs directly. If a person has worked successfully at re-evaluating negative automatic thoughts, both in sessions and in vivo, then very often there is an automatic re-appraisal of the more general beliefs, particularly at the level of dysfunctional assumptions. Even so, one shouldn't assume this so always ask about new rules for living and new general perspectives before discharge.

Agnes had strong beliefs about never expressing anger. In a range of situations, she experimented with being more assertive, including in situations where people were behaving unreasonably. During debriefing of her experiences it became clear that her beliefs about expressing anger were modified, although they were not directly addressed.

To help your patient become their own therapist reflect closely on what is taking place in therapy. Ask questions such as 'What were we doing there?', 'Can you identify the kind of skewed thinking you had there?', 'How could you use that strategy in other situations?' It is important that you attribute progress to the patient's efforts, particularly if they are at risk of attributing change to your attention and skill rather than their own.

As treatment progresses, the frequency of sessions may be reduced, perhaps moving to two-weekly, followed by perhaps a three- or four-week break before treatment ends.

ENDING THERAPY

The end of therapy is a handover of responsibility from you to your patient. Aim for your patient to be skilled enough to:

- continue to progress towards unmet (realistic) goals and
- manage their own setbacks.

It is crucial to review relapse management skills and it is time to develop a *blueprint* for dealing with problems that may emerge in the future.

Blueprints

A blueprint is an aide-memoire, a reminder of vulnerabilities, strengths and coping strategies, that is constructed towards the end of therapy. It complements the skill of relapse management training (Chapter 9).

Blueprints generally contain the following:

- An understanding of the problem(s): a parsimonious reminder of personal 'traps' and vulnerabilities.
- Helpful coping strategies.
- Situations that may be difficult, or could possibly lead to a recurrence of the problem.
- Ways of responding to this.

Most worksheets are best tailored to the individual and need to be devised with the patient. Below are two examples of blueprints and you can see that they cover essentially the same areas of information but that each patient uses different wording, order and emphasis (see Figure 4.2). A personalised blueprint will have more validity and then there is more chance that it will be used.

Discharge

At discharge a long-term management 'kit' would usefully comprise:

- the *skill* of relapse management (see Chapter 9)
- a blueprint
- a positive formulation – a reminder of strengths and assets (see Chapter 5).

Dominique: Overcoming my urge to self-harm	
I am at risk when...	My mood gets low I drink Someone upsets me
Early warning signs ...	I withdraw Get irritable Start drinking alone
What I can do to stop myself	Don't keep blades in the house Contact friends Drink soda Put in my ear buds and watch videos on-line Use my soothing images and relaxation exercises Remind myself of all the reasons for not harming (Keep my list on my phone)
Damage limitation if I harm	Text friend asap! Only use clean blades and put antiseptic cream on the cuts Go to my diary and try to understand what's going on and why. I can learn from this.
Bart: Managing my depression	
What I've learnt during therapy	"I understand that my depression stemmed from a cluster of stressful events and the final straw was my job change. I now know that I get caught in traps of negative thinking and inactivity – but I can break free of them and then my mood improves."
Helpful strategies	"Avoiding getting over stressed: plan ahead. Using thought records or distraction to break the negative thinking trap. Getting active asap."
When I'll be at risk of setback	"When I get stressed and have thoughts like: 'I can't cope, everything will collapse round my ears,' my mood worsens, and I close down mentally and physically."
Ways of responding	"Think what I'd say to a friend in a similar position; look at my log of recent situations where I tackled difficulties (including getting a new job, coping with my wife's unexpected illness); talk with my wife and friends; start walking to and from work again."

Figure 4.2   Examples of blueprints

It is relatively easy to work towards ending therapy if you share the notion that treatment is finite, and you regularly review goals and progress.

Rather than having an abrupt end to treatment, you might plan a follow-up or booster session or two over the subsequent year. You can continue to review progress, reinforce successes, review how problems are managed, spot re-emergences of unhelpful patterns of thinking or behaviour, and work together to troubleshoot if necessary.

Despite the gradual withdrawal from therapy, and the emphasis on skills acquisition, some people do worry that they will not cope independently. Tackle this in a standard CBT way, by identifying and reviewing worrying thoughts – perhaps supporting this with relevant experiments.

Measures, such as questionnaires or self-monitoring indices, should be administered at the end of therapy. The outcome of CBT with most of your patients is likely to be good. However, some will not have benefited from treatment, and this can be especially difficult for those who came to cognitive therapy having had little success with other treatment approaches. Ideally, poor progress is identified at an early stage, so that CBT can be ended sooner rather than later, but whenever it is discontinued consider that cognitive therapy has not delivered, rather than the patient has failed.

'Although we have developed an understanding of why you might have your difficulties and you have given CBT a reasonable trial, it does seem that it has not made much difference to your problems. CBT doesn't meet everyone's needs and sometimes the timing is just not right. I think at this point we have to say that CBT is not delivering what you need. Perhaps we should look at what has been useful, so that you can take away some strategies for helping you feel better. For example, we found that you were good at breaking problems down into different elements, and that you could then tackle difficult situations more easily. We can also review the formulation that we drew up together and rethink about what therapeutic approach might better meet your needs.'

While it may be difficult to end treatment when there has been little gain, it is unfair to maintain false hopes. If it seems that a different approach would be more useful, discuss this as early on as possible: for example, if there are significant relationship problems that obstruct CBT then couples therapy, or possibly systemic therapy, could be suggested; or it may be worth considering medication if this has not been tried. Whenever discharge occurs, developing a blueprint along with a positive formulation (see Chapter 5) if possible, ends treatment on a hopeful note.

Mutual feedback

Throughout treatment we should be sharing feedback but at the end of therapy it is particularly important to:

- elicit from patients ways in which CBT and you as a therapist met their needs and gather their suggestions for improvement – not only can this information be reviewed to refine your own practice, but it can also prompt your patients to consider what this might tell them about effective self-help;

- feedback to patients the ways in which they used therapy to best advantage and reinforce learning and achievements that might otherwise be unappreciated – then explore how they can build on this in their independent coping.

Of course, some of this work will have been done in the context of blueprinting.

Time-limited CBT

As we know, CBT was intended as a time-limited and focused intervention. Some of us might find that our service demands that we deliver very time-limited therapy indeed, perhaps to the extent that we feel unable to offer an appropriate intervention. On the other hand, some of us might work in systems that impose no limits. Both situations need to be given thought.

Working with limited sessions

Since the instigation of Improving Access to Psychological Therapies (IAPT: Department of Health, 2007), there has been a system in place in England and Wales for evaluating the impact of relatively brief, focused CBT. IAPT presents very clear guidelines for therapists who work within a well-defined stepped-care framework. Similar boundaries might usefully operate elsewhere, for example within private organisations where the length and type of intervention are dictated by insurance companies.

The *Low Intensity* (LI) phase of IAPT offers computerised CBT, guided self-help, psychoeducational groups, behavioural activation, while the *High Intensity* (HI) step comprises traditional CBT for non-complex psychological problems.

One of the many strengths of IAPT is the clarity of guidance for working at each step and another is conscientious outcome data collection. The data from IAPT reviews has been illuminating and might well have relevance for other services and practitioners (see Layard & Clark, 2014 for a review). In summary, the best rates of recovery were when:

- there was good fidelity to the empirically recommended CBT approach;
- therapists were more experienced/more highly trained;
- patients received more sessions (for a 50% recovery rate, an average of eight or more sessions was required in many services);
- there was good referral on to more specialist services when initial interventions proved insufficient;
- NICE guidelines were closely followed.

Thus, a relatively brief intervention can be effective if we are conscientious about developing therapist competency and respecting treatment fidelity and patient need. At an OCTC Congress in 2015 Professor David Clark, one of the main instigators of IAPT, made a plea that IAPT interventions be guided by patient-sensitive CBT formulation, and that patients receive the level of therapy that they need not an arbitrary number of sessions dictated by a service. Sound advice.

Offering long-term interventions

There is no doubt that some patients need more sessions than others and again Professor Clark's appeal to formulate sensitively is relevant. Once engaged in CBT, people are likely to need longer if they have:

- complex presenting problems (because of chronicity, co-morbidity or co-existing personality disorder) and
- poor resources (*inner resources* such as good problem-solving skills or *external resources* such as social support).

Your formulation will give you insights into this and will direct therapy – if CBT is suitable for your patient. Remember that virtually all presenting problems can be formulated but not everyone is ready for CBT.

It is sometimes absolutely necessary to invest additional time in engaging and treating a patient, but this must be kept under close review. Progress towards clear goals should be scrutinised (possibly every five to ten sessions). You can do a disservice to patients by not discharging those who are ready to experience independence or by not referring on those whose needs could be better met elsewhere.

SUMMARY

- A course of CBT has a clear arc of early, later and ending stages.
- The early stages are particularly active in engaging and preparing patients for therapy.
- The later stages emphasise gaining confidence and independent coping skills and the therapist is actively judging how long to continue the work.
- Ending therapy is a carefully orchestrated phase where coping skills for life are fine-tuned.
- Throughout, attention is paid to the therapeutic relationship, relapse management, skill development.

REFLECTION & ACTION

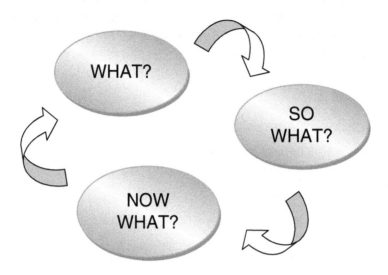

WHAT are you taking away from this chapter? What teaching points resonate with you?

....

....

....

....

....

....

....

....

....

....

SO WHAT? What significance do these points have – how do they relate to your previous learning or views? Do they challenge your former opinions? Have you gleaned new ideas for helping patients or indeed looking after your own needs?

....

....

....

....

....

....

....

....

....

....

NOW WHAT? How will you now address structuring a course of CBT? What are you now going to do differently? Make a commitment with yourself to follow through on at least one of your new ideas.

....

....

....

....

....

....

....

....

....

....

5

FORMULATING PROBLEMS

Assessment and formulation is CBT's chicken and egg. We do have to assess before we can formulate a person's problems, but we must first have a sound understanding of formulation to guide our enquiries and define our provisional conclusions. We need to hold in mind a generic framework of formulation *alongside* established models as both help us develop the hypotheses that we check out in our assessment.

Therefore, a good starting point is the framework that underpins CBT – the formulation (also referred to as the conceptualisation).

FORMULATIONS

Formulations are personal representations of problem(s) that explain why a person developed difficulties and, most importantly, why they are not going away. There is a widely accepted generic framework used to understand this in CBT and there are many problem-specific models, empirically tailored to particular difficulties. Beck tells us to start with the generic (Beck & Haigh, 2014).

The generic formulation

Our first widely-used framework was the model of depression proposed by Beck et al. (1979). This captured psychological processes that were common across psychological problems and so it proved to be an adaptable template that was soon applied to other psychological disorders. Thus, Beck's early framework came to represent a broad structure for understanding

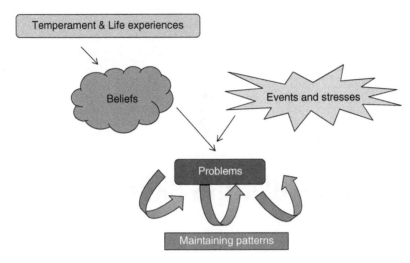

Figure 5.1 Simple generic formulation

psychological difficulties, capturing maintaining patterns, and setting up hypotheses to be tested. As Beck says, 'The generic cognitive model represents a set of common principles that can be applied across the spectrum of psychological disorders' (Beck & Haigh, 2014: 1–24).

A simple generic formulation, based on Beck's idea, is set out in Figure 5.1. More about simple CBT formulations can be downloaded from the OCTC website at www.octc.co.uk/wp-content/uploads/2016/04/OCTC-Clinical-Innovations-Blobby-formulation-Final-April-2016.pdf.

In some cases, simply arriving at a formulation will be therapeutic because it will help a patient understand that it is no wonder that they developed the problem and it will illustrate possibilities for change. This alone can sometimes shift key beliefs and give relief, but more often than not there is more work to be done.

In short, developing a formulation should do several things:

- Explain why a problem persists.
- Explain why a person developed the problem in the first place.
- Educate the patient about the cognitive model and CBT.
- Strengthen our therapeutic alliance.

The maintaining cycles: why don't problems go away?

Arguably, the most crucial aspects of the formulation are the maintaining cycles, or the 'traps' that people fall into, because these give us the focus of treatment. Sometimes this is all we need to use in our conceptualisation because a detailed historical background is not relevant.

Once we have identified unhelpful patterns of thoughts and behaviours we can use our wealth of CBT strategies to help patients learn how to break free of these traps.

In CBT, we look for the interaction of the cognitions, behaviours, emotions and physical reactions that drive problems. Within specific disorders there are some quite particular patterns (e.g. catastrophic thinking and hyperventilation driving panic cycles), but there are also common patterns across disorders. Harvey et al. (2004) explored these in their text on cognitive-behavioural processes across psychological disorders and their book is well worth a read. Some of the most predominant processes are explored below.

Emotional drivers

Probably the most common emotional maintaining factor is relief, at least in the short term. For example, a fearful person will feel immediate respite on gaining reassurance or deciding not to face the fear, someone with an urge to binge or to self-injure might feel good as soon as they give themself permission to over-eat or hurt themselves, while a furious person may have an immediate satisfying sense of release on lashing out. That relief is often short-lived however, and the individual will not have had a successful experience of managing their problem. Not surprisingly then, the problem will remain in place (see Figure 5.2).

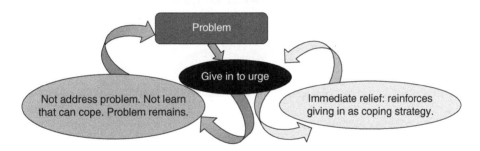

Figure 5.2 Emotionally-driven maintaining cycle

Behavioural drivers

The behavioural driver at the heart of many persistent difficulties is often (but not exclusively) avoidance and escape:

Jay had feared spiders for as long as he could remember. His immediate thoughts were 'they will crawl on me and I can't bear the idea!' This fueled his fear and he avoided going anywhere where he might see them. In this way he did not have to face his fear but, and this is the crucial bit, he never learnt that he might be able to tolerate spiders. His prediction stayed intact – as did his fear.

When Kay got low, she believed that she would be awful company: 'No-one would want to be with me and I can't face the humiliation of rejection.' Predictably, she avoided social contact and if she found herself with people she exited as soon as possible. This meant that she became more isolated and in turn this robbed her of social confidence and the isolation lowered her mood.

Although his friends told him that he looked good, Lance believed that he was unattractive and overweight. He avoided looking in mirrors and he wore shapeless hooded tops that hid his body and, if necessary, his face. In doing so he got immediate relief: 'I/people can't see how fat and ugly I am.' But this meant that he never saw for himself that he looked normal and when friends reassured him, he didn't believe them because he believed that he had hidden his true appearance from them.

It is evident from these examples that avoidance backfires (see Figure 5.3) and that's what we are looking for in maintaining cycles – the trap that stops the problem resolving.

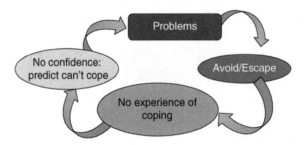

Figure 5.3 Avoidance-driven maintaining cycle

Cognitive drivers

Possibly the most commonly cited cognitive 'trap' is driven by 'safety-seeking behaviours' (SSBs) (Salkovskis, Clark, & Gelder, 1996). You might wonder why a 'behaviour' is in a cognitive category. This is because an SSB is determined by a person's *interpretation* of a behaviour, it does not refer to a behaviour per se.

For example, recently I decided to distract myself to be more at ease during a dental procedure. I reckoned that I could tolerate the uncomfortable procedure – but why suffer unnecessarily when I could make things more bearable for myself? Things went smoothly and the experience left me feeling in control and more confident about facing similar procedures in the future. Now, compare this to someone in the same situation, using the same strategy but interpreting the outcome quite differently. If their interpretation were 'Thank goodness I used distraction – that's what got me through, I wouldn't have managed without it ...', then they might well feel less confident in the longer term. Instead of believing that they can cope, they predict that they can only manage by using distraction. They continue to rely on it and they develop a powerful SSB that they dare not drop (see Figure 5.4).

Other common cognitively-driven traps were identified in Chapter 1: exaggerated thinking; self-reproachful thinking; negative thinking; intuitive thinking. Selective attention is another common driver, e.g. the person with low self-esteem who only notices criticisms and not praise, the person with health anxiety who scans their body and notices discomforts that they interpret as illness, the person with a spider phobia who selectively notes anything that could indicate the presence of a spider ('Fruit bowl – there could be spiders in there! Faint crack in the plaster – or it could be a spider web! Random marks on the paintwork – could be spider droppings!').

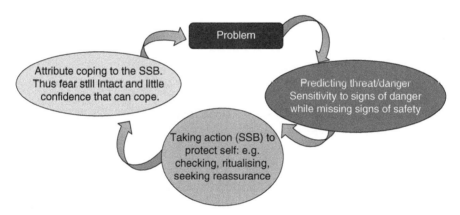

Figure 5.4 Cognitively-driven maintaining cycle

Detailing the maintaining cycles

The more detail we have in the cycles, the more opportunities there are for identifying ways of breaking free. You can use your skills of Socratic enquiry and monitoring (see Chapters 7 and 8) to gather the detailed information you need to make sense of the persistence of a problem.

The detailed elements of the maintaining cycle tell us what interventions are relevant. When we have identified relevant emotional components, we can consider mood managing strategies; we can help patients deal with behavioural mechanisms through practical experiments and we can coach patients in cognitive techniques to combat the cognitive components. By sharing this message with our patients – the message that we can spot the cause and match a solution – we are communicating hope. Hope improves prognosis and helps cement our working alliance.

Why did this person develop these problems?

Although the maintaining cycle is where most of the CBT-action is, it can be helpful also to consider why a person developed a particular problem in the first place. In general, problems come about because of the way we think (and behave) in response to events:

Alec had never had many friends and he believed that he was dull, so when his friend left the area without a proper goodbye, he took this as proof that he was not worth bothering with and his mood worsened.

Britta had always been a bit of a worrier and when the demands of being a single mother grew, she found herself getting more stressed and anxious about all sorts of things. Her GP said she had GAD.

Cal had always been told that he was special and given most of what he'd asked for. Understandably he felt that he should have his own way, so when his new boss began to challenge Cal's views and refuse his requests, he lost his temper – frequently.

In these examples, the interplay of each person's inner world with life events and stresses was a recipe for misery, anxiety or anger, so it's *no wonder* that Alec, Britta and Cal developed problems (see Figure 5.5). Once we can share 'It's no wonder ...' we communicate a non-judgmental empathy, and as we already know this enhances our therapeutic alliance.

We can then help our patients appreciate why their difficulties are understandable, and in doing so provide relevant psychoeducation. And there is more – we are now aware of their psychological vulnerabilities so we can check that these have changed by the end of treatment. It is crucial to do this because without change there is a greater risk of setbacks. If Alec continues to believe that he is dull (even if his friend returns) or if Britta's stress levels remain high (even if she becomes less of a worrier) they will be vulnerable to relapse.

Once you have shared an understanding of the origin of the problem, it's time to shift the emphasis to the here and now. You will find yourself referring back every now and then,

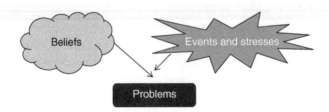

Figure 5.5   Problems developing from interplay of beliefs and events

keeping the problem in context, but in CBT the active work focuses on the maintaining cycles.

The positive formulation

Several CBT practitioners have advocated developing a positive, functional framework to guide long-term coping (e.g. Kuyken et al., 2009; Layden, Newman, Freeman & Morse, 1993). There are several reasons to consider this.

Recognising current strengths and assets

Noting a patient's resources can provide a constructive balance and help keep problems in perspective. It is not unusual for patients to have a 'blind sight' for their skills, talents and assets, so the therapist needs to be on the lookout for them and able to depict achievements and strengths in a constructive conceptualisation.

When prompted and given time, Cassie was able to recall a person who had been kind and encouraging. From Year 6–8 her schoolteacher, Ms Bellock, had understood Cassie's struggle with reading and was patient. She had seen Cassie's musical abilities and had encouraged her to play guitar in the after-school club. From this Cassie learnt that some people are kind and that she was smart and had talents. When she dwelt on this she felt safer and more confident, and in that frame of mind and with that emotional state she was more likely to brave social situations. Once she began to go out more her social confidence grew, and she got caught up in a virtuous cycle.

Recording progress

As a patient develops more coping strategies, a positive formulation can capture and reinforce progress. Thus, a formulation should be under constant review and as vicious cycles are tackled, the new virtuous cycles need to be recorded. These conceptualisations then form a guide and reminder of what works for the patient, and as such are an essential part of coping in the long term.

Considering possibilities

Padesky (in Kuyken et al., 2009) advocates a third type of positive formulation, one of possibilities. She encourages patients to consider *what could be* and what needs to be in place (in terms of thoughts and behaviours) to make this happen. She might take the patient's goal of 'being more socially confident' and help her patient detail what this will look like, how it might feel, what thoughts the patient would have, and what behaviours would be seen. This would then form a constructive framework to guide the patient towards what they could achieve.

Some people find it easier to be guided by the 'can do' framework of a positive formulation rather than always striving to avoid getting caught up in pathological patterns, but this is something to explore with your patient, of course.

Disorder specific models and formulations

Although the generic framework proposes that many clinical disorders share common under-lying processes, various disorders can now be reliably distinguished by the content of beliefs and characteristic behaviours. Over time specific models have been developed to capture the particular aetiological and maintaining factors for particular problems. Some of these are rela-tively simple maintaining patterns, such as Clark's elegant (1986) panic model, while others include more neuro-psychological, behavioural and physiological elements, such as Ehlers and Clark's (2000) PTSD model. Many of the models have been rigorously evaluated, but you do need to be aware that sometimes the term 'model' is used to describe a theoretical idea that has not yet gathered empirical support and these will not be as compelling, for example Kirk and Rouf's very well considered but untested (2004) model of specific phobia.

Aim to make yourself familiar with these various diagnostic heuristics as you will need this knowledge to inform your own conceptualisations. Table 5.1 summarises some of the

Table 5.1 Prominent CBT models

Specific Disorder	
Depression	Beck et al. (1979)
Specific phobia	Kirk & Rouf (2004)
Panic disorder and agoraphobia	Clark (1986); Wells (1997)
Health anxiety	Salkovskis & Warwick (1986); Warwick & Salkovskis (1989)
Social anxiety	Clark (2002); Clark & Wells (1995); Wells (1997)
Generalised anxiety disorder (GAD)	Borkovec & Newman (1999); Borkovec et al. (2002); Wells (1997, 2000)
Obsessive-compulsive disorder (OCD)	Salkovskis (1985, 1999); Wells (1997)
Post-traumatic stress disorder (PTSD)	Ehlers & Clark (2000)
Eating disorders (transdiagnostic)	Waller (1993); Fairburn et al. (2003)
Anger	Novaco (1979); Beck & Fernandez (1998)
Psychosis	Garety et al. (2001); Morrison (2001); Tarrier & Haddock (2002)
Bi-polar disorder	Scott (1996); Mansell et al. (2005)

most prominent of the well-established models and you will see that many are reassuringly longstanding.

Beck and Haigh (2014) propose beginning CBT with a generic framework to guide the assessment but advise continually asking – is this understanding of my patient's problems mapping onto recognised models? If the answer is 'no', then we can continue to use Beck's generic framework to formulate and to develop ideas about interventions. If the answer is 'yes' then we can populate the pre-existing model with our patient's experiences, thus transforming a theoretical framework into a personal formulation.

Nadia had a vomit phobia, for which there is no well-established, empirically-based cognitive model. Her therapist used the generic framework to shape a formulation, which revealed that it was understandable that Nadia had developed her fear. She had always been repelled by vomit, the sight and smell of it made her nauseous, but as a teenager she had been violently sick when out with friends. She had felt ashamed and there was a moment when she thought that she might choke to death. Her current beliefs were: 'If I see or smell vomit I will be violently sick and out of control. I can't bear the sensation. I will be judged by people and feel ashamed. I must protect myself from seeing vomit or risking being sick.' This understanding was sufficient for Nadia to accept that it was no wonder that she had developed her fear – but why didn't it just go away? The answer was that there were many vicious cycles (or traps) that fueled the fear, and one by one she and her therapist teased out the detail of each.

Emotional relief: Once she had decided that she was not going to put herself at risk of seeing vomit or being sick, she would feel a wave of relief, which was reinforcing (see Figure 5.6).

Avoidance: She avoided going out so that she would not risk seeing vomit in the street. This meant that she never learnt that she could tolerate being outside or that she could tolerate seeing vomit (see Figure 5.6).

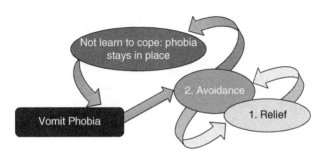

Figure 5.6   Nadia's Avoidance trap

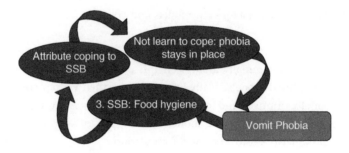

Figure 5.7 Nadia's SSB trap

SSB: She was overly conscientious about food hygiene. When she was not sick, she attributed this to her careful preparation of food and so she continued to maintain very high standards of hygiene, afraid of letting her standards drop (see Figure 5.7).

Looking out for danger signs: Nadia was hypersensitive to signs of danger and as a result would scan for and notice any sign of vomit. She also often mistook innocent things as threatening, for example mistaking bird droppings for vomit. As a result, her fears of being confronted by vomit when she was outdoors stayed in place (see Figure 5.8).

Panic: Exploring the hypervigilance trap revealed a pattern reminiscent of Clark's panic model. If Nadia thought she was in danger, catastrophic thoughts of vomiting without being able to stop (or choking on her vomit) filled her mind. She feared the humiliation of this and she had fleeting fears

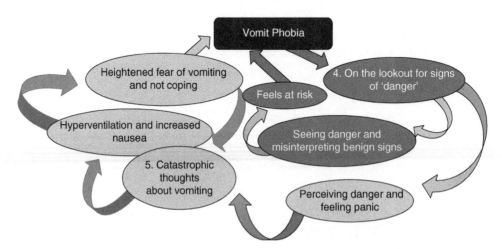

Figure 5.8 Nadia's Hypervigilance and Panic trap

of death. Understandably this fueled feelings of panic, and then she hyperventilated, felt even more nauseous and panicked more. Although she did not fulfil the diagnostic criteria for panic disorder, her experience closely mapped onto Clark's panic model and this became a relevant heuristic that guided formulating that aspect of her problem and generated ideas for intervention (see Figure 5.8).

Although specifics are important in understanding maintaining patterns, a formulation with details of all the vicious cycles is too complicated, especially for a patient who is just learning about CBT. So a first step might be to simplify each cycle (see Figure 5.9) and then to isolate, detail and address each one at a time. This simple but sophisticated representation of a problem is often called a 'Vicious Flower' (see Butler et al., 2008 for a comprehensive description of both vicious and virtuous flowers).

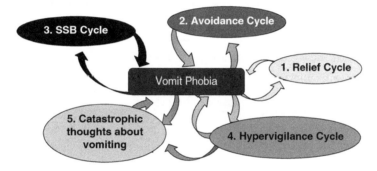

Figure 5.9 Nadia's maintaining cycles for vomit phobia

Each unhelpful pattern tells us what needs to be done in therapy: fears that need to be faced, behaviours to change, cognitions to be addressed and so on. In the case of Nadia, cycles 1–4 could be addressed using first principles of CBT, while managing cycle 5 would be informed by Clark's panic protocol (1986).

But we are getting ahead of ourselves – first we need to review how we gather the information needed to develop these detailed and personalised understandings of why problems don't go away. This takes us into the next chapter on assessment, which is our opportunity for gathering a range of information including positive details, such as are illustrated in Figures 5.10 and 5.11.

Nadia also had times of coping (which she often overlooked). She and her therapist identified one time recently when she had managed to control her anxiety about vomit. From this she recognised that staying and checking out her predictions paid off (see Figure 5.10).

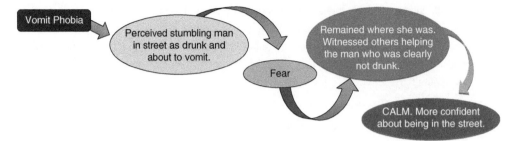

Figure 5.10   Nadia's coping cycles for vomit phobia

There were also times when she had coped with other fears and reviewing these helped her appreciate that she had some good coping strategies that she might later apply to managing her vomit phobia. For example, she could recall some successful experiences of facing the fear and using encouraging self-talk (which then set up virtuous cycles of increasing confidence).

One situation where Nadia had coped well was in the park with her small nephew. A dog had approached them and Nadia had not wanted to show fear in front of her nephew so she acted as if she were calm. She consciously tried to relax and kept her voice and posture composed. Although she didn't want to encourage him to approach a strange dog, she commented that the dog was pretty and friendly and they looked at it from a distance. She discovered that she was actually becoming more relaxed and believing what she told her nephew about the dog being friendly and there being nothing to worry about. This reinforced her confidence that she could face her fears (see Figure 5.11).

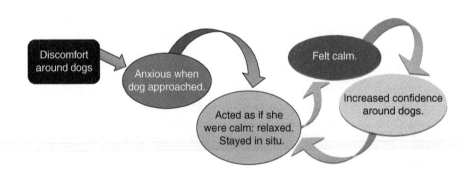

Figure 5.11   Nadia's coping cycles for dog phobia

Using your formulation(s)

If you and your patient are to get the most out of the formulation a few guidelines are worth considering:

Evolve and share, don't prepare and present A formulation represents the patient's inner world and experiences. Therapists simply bring along the theory to guide and shape an understanding. You can only be confident that a formulation captures a patient's reality if you build it up together. This also achieves the goal of teaching the skill of self-formulation, a skill that will be needed if patients are to become independent.

Keep it as simple as you can Yes, you will need to embrace enough detail for a person to be able to relate to the conceptualisation but try not to go much beyond this. Too complicated a framework can confuse and overwhelm.

Keep it updated A formulation is a snapshot of where a patient is now and it remains your best guide for intervention. If therapy has an impact, then the formulation should be changing to accommodate this. If the patient's experiences change (such as getting a new job, ending a relationship, improved mood) then this needs to be reflected in the conceptualisation. Your revised formulation can then help you refine your interventions.

SUMMARY

- CBT formulations bring together theory and clinical reality.
- They explain why a person might have developed a problem and clarify the maintaining patterns that hinder recovery.
- The problem-maintaining cycles inform appropriate treatment plans.
- Coping patterns can also contribute to treatment.
- Some formulations are founded on a generic understanding of psychological problems, while others are based on problem-specific models – but a formulation should always be personal to your patient.
- A 'good' formulation is shared and updated in line with changes in the patient's experiences.

REFLECTION & ACTION

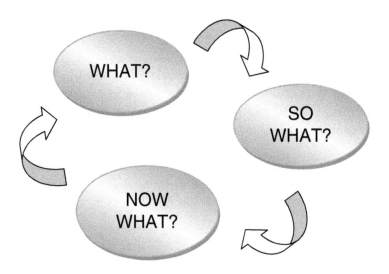

WHAT are you taking away from this chapter? What teaching points resonate with you?

....

....

....

....

....

....

....

....

....

SO WHAT? What significance do these points have – how do they relate to your previous learning or views? Do they challenge your former opinions? Have you gleaned new ideas for helping patients or indeed looking after your own needs?

....

....

....

....

....

....

....

....

....

....

NOW WHAT? How will you now address formulating your patient's problem? What are you now going to do differently? Make a commitment with yourself to follow through on at least one of your new ideas.

....

....

....

....

....

....

....

....

....

....

6

ASSESSING PROBLEMS

The aim of a CBT assessment is to amass the information that we need to develop a shared formulation. It is a systematic process shaped by the formulation frameworks described in the previous chapter. However, assessment demands more than following a checklist of key questions. It is a sensitive, reactive and flexible process that respects and strengthens your therapeutic alliance. Within this, hypotheses are developed and explored, and to get the most from assessment, your patient needs to be engaged and motivated (see Chapter 2).

STRUCTURING ASSESSMENT

The process

The process of assessment is summarised in Figure 6.1. You can see that it begins with gathering information (and this will already be influenced by hypotheses that you have about the presenting problem and about the general and demographic information that will be relevant).

If we hold in mind general and problem-specific conceptualisations of difficulties, we can review a patient's responses in the light of these and then refine our hunches about what makes sense of this person's problems. This might require us to gather more information and gradually we will build up a database that might well explain why this person has these difficulties and why they are persistent.

With much reflection and tweaking we progress towards a shared understanding with our patient. At first this working formulation might be simple, a modest vicious cycle for example,

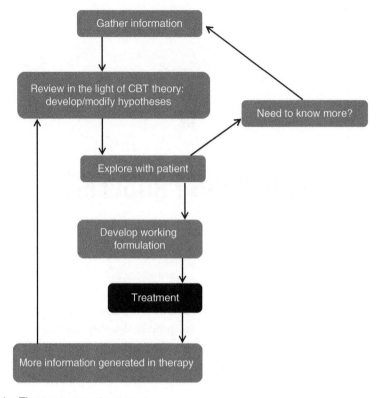

Figure 6.1 The assessment process

but it will often build into something more comprehensive such as a framework that also captures the origin and precipitant of a problem.

Once the formulation seems to make sense of the situation it will give us ideas for treatment – but assessment doesn't stop there. A good formulation is dynamic, it changes as circumstances change, and as such assessment is ongoing.

What do I need to know?

Essentially you need to discover answers to the following questions.

How does this patient experience the problem?

What are the cognitions, feelings, behaviours and physical sensations? These can be teased out and patterns revealed. As you collect this information try to link the steps together to understand what vicious cycle(s) might be at the heart of the problem.

'I know that you've described your difficulties to a few people by now, but it would be really helpful if I could hear what the problem is in your own words. Would that be okay?'

- I'm scared most of the time, physically tense, and I try to avoid people as much as possible. I feel stupid and I think that people can see this, and they despise me. They are going to humiliate me.
- I don't really feel much, just leaden and hopeless. When I'm alone with my own thoughts, I sit and vegetate. I keep thinking 'Loser' and I can't get going.
- I want to lose weight, but I get hungry then I eat some junk and then I hate myself. Then I eat (and drink) for comfort but end up feeling dreadful and determined to diet the next day.

What sets it off?

It is unlikely that someone suffers at the same level all day, every day, so find out what triggers the problem (and later what contextual factors make a difference to its severity). Look out for situational, social, cognitive, physiological, affective and behavioural variables as these can each play a vital part in linking vicious cycles.

'What's likely to trigger the problem? Any particular places or events?'

- Going out and being amongst people (or even thinking about it) triggers real panic. That's the worst.
- Whenever I'm alone I power down, put things off and waste time.
- Being hungry triggers eating and as soon as I've started to eat junk, I think I've blown it, so I keep going. Drinking alcohol makes me more likely to overeat or eat junk food – so does being anxious or stressed.

Some patients experience their problems as being the same all the time, always there. This might be so, but we need to check it out because if there are times of fluctuation, we can build on them to maximise periods of respite. Asking a patient to keep a log can help them monitor, say, hourly variations. This can then help address the next enquiry.

What makes a difference?

To properly understand patterns, we need to know what eases the problem and what exacerbates it.

'Is there anything that makes the problem worse? Anything that eases it?'

- Being with someone I trust or going to a familiar place makes it easier. New places and being alone make it harder.
- Being with a friend and doing something makes me feel a bit better but it never lasts. If I'm at home alone, Facetime with a friend can make it easier or finding a task that I must do.
- If I have a structured day it helps and if I've prepared food in advance, I'm less likely to eat junk even when I get hungry and need to eat.

Medication (prescribed or otherwise) might be relevant here, so don't forget to ask about that.

What's the upshot?

The final part of our investigation is what happens as a result of the problems. The general questions to consider are:

'What impact has this problem had on your life? How has life changed because of the problem?'

'How have others (friends, family, doctors, work colleagues, etc.) responded to the problem?'

'What coping strategies have you tried, and how successful were they?'

- I just don't go out much and I miss so many opportunities. I don't socialise, I don't go for jobs. I'm ashamed of myself and then I'm even less self-confident.
- I get more tired – and more hopeless about being back at work. Then it's even harder to do things. People have started to give up on me and I'm getting lonelier.
- I've tried restricting myself, but it always backfires.

As we gather information in these four areas (the problem, the triggers, what makes a difference and the upshot), we see how thoughts, feelings and behaviours interplay and we can start to build up an understanding of a particular problem and why it isn't going away: a maintenance formulation.

Why me?

Sometimes a maintenance level of understanding is enough to help our patients, but sometimes it is beneficial to learn more of the origins of a problem. It is relatively easy to ask questions about a person's history and hypothesise about vulnerability factors, but remember to be sensitive to signs of discomfort in your patient.

We know that certain experiences render a person vulnerable to particular problems, e.g. Brown and Harris's classic (1978) work showed us that childhood loss of a parent increases vulnerability to depression, and we know from psychological trauma research that experiencing a significant traumatic event increases the likelihood of PTSD. However, this does not mean that *everyone* who has lost a parent or suffered a trauma will inevitably become depressed or develop PTSD. For problems to develop other events need to come into play, and so assessment needs to be broad-ranging enough to establish why it really is understandable that our patient suffers their particular difficulties.

'It might help me to understand a bit more about the background to this problem and why you developed it in the first place. Is it alright if I ask some questions about your past? Do tell me if you feel uncomfortable at any time – we can always move on to something else.'

- I can't remember a time when I felt safe around people. Mum was so poorly during my childhood I didn't feel that I had anywhere to turn and I was bullied at school and the teachers gave me a hard time because of my dyslexia so I became afraid of everybody. I can see why I now expect to be humiliated and why I hide away whenever I can.
- I thought that if I was good enough, we would be a happy family, that my parents would stop fighting and would stop taking it out on us, too. Nothing changed and I always felt ashamed that I wasn't good enough. I kept myself to myself for years, bottling up all these thoughts and feelings. I coped quite well until I lost my job and then it all came to the surface – no wonder it feels like too much to handle now.
- I joined a gym at university for fun but my friends got so serious and body conscious that for the first time ever I began to worry about the way my body looked. When someone I'd fancied called me 'gym blob' I starved myself to get thinner. I kept it up for about a month, lost 20 pounds and then binged at a drunken party. That's when my problem began.

This sort of exploration helps us address the common question: 'Why me?' Then we can genuinely conclude that it really is no wonder that a person developed a problem.

TOOLS AT MY DISPOSAL

We have several means of gathering information to help us properly understand a patient's difficulties: direct questions, Socratic enquiry, formal assessments, and bespoke measures.

Whatever the choice of appraisal there is never a right or wrong answer, and however a patient responds it is cause for curiosity. Let your patients know this so they don't freeze with performance anxiety.

Direct questions

These are ideal for straightforward data collection: How do you feel? What do you do? What do you weigh? Do you have thoughts of killing yourself? How often does this happen? Are there times when it is easier for you? What is the worst situation? It goes without saying that such questions need to be asked sensitively.

Socratic enquiry and Socratic method

We can often elicit an even better understanding by helping a person reflect on their own knowledge and experience by asking questions that prompt reflection or setting up self-monitoring that will reveal useful information. These Socratic approaches are elaborated in Chapter 7 and 8, so they aren't covered in detail here.

Formal measures

There are many questionnaires and checklists available to the cognitive therapist. Some are free to use while others need to be purchased. The most important distinction is that some have good psychometric properties and others don't. When standardised instruments are developed, attention is usually paid to *validity* and *reliability*. Aim to use measures with robust validity and reliability.

A *valid* measure measures what it says it measures and not some irrelevant feature, e.g. a social anxiety questionnaire should measure just that, and not be so complex that responses to it are affected by a person's verbal ability, or so off beam that it also targets agoraphobia.

A *reliable* measure is repeatable, it achieves the same result or score when repeated under the same conditions at another time, or with another assessor. A measure low in reliability produces inconsistent findings.

Bespoke measures

These are measures that we create and usually tailor to the patient. You will find some standard templates in the final section of this book and there are other examples in academic papers, books and on the internet. You can also easily devise simple and personalised measures with your patient. These might include the following.

Frequency counts

Counting is a simple and reliable method that can assess the frequency of many things: ATS; checking; repetitive behaviours; handwipes used; phone calls made/received; angry outbursts;

urges to binge. The target is determined by your patient's need. However, it is often helpful to avoid lengthy recording of something that has a very high rate as this is too demanding. Instead, ask the patient to take a sample at a meaningful time of day, e.g. a half-hour period when the problem is prominent. If there is no reason to focus on a particular time, opt for an arbitrary time.

Duration of events

The duration of an event or experience may also be relevant and easily monitored. Examples include time spent washing or body checking or travelling alone or binge-eating or concentrating on a task. Again, the possibilities are endless but they should always be pertinent to the patient.

Self-ratings and personalised logs

These can capture even more information about behaviours, emotions and cognitions. For example, patients can be asked to rate several pieces of information, such as what they are doing, when and how they feel. They can detail this by using a rating scale and log. Two logs in common use are described later: Thought Records (Chapter 7) and Activity Schedules (Chapter 8). The logs must always be tailored to a patient's needs and abilities – check that your patients can understand relevant written instructions and don't over-tax them. It is always a good idea to practise completing a log together in the session.

Information collected over a period of time can be collated, e.g. weekly mood ratings or strength of belief can be usefully represented in a graph. Not only does such a collection of data show progress but fluctuations in data can also be readily linked with events.

Alejandro struggled with long-standing low self-esteem. However, when he and his therapist graphed his weekly ratings on a standardised self-esteem questionnaire, they could see a general improvement in his ratings over a three-month period. There were, however, two dips that were linked to visits from his [critical] ex-partner. This visual evidence buoyed up Alejandro because he had been underestimating his progress, but it also reminded him that he was still vulnerable to setback when criticised. He and his therapist then devised a plan to target this interpersonal challenge.

Whatever your choice of measure, remember that observations made at the time are more reliable than retrospective estimates (Barlow, Hayes & Nelson, 1984).

'I would have sworn that I felt bad all of the time and it was only when I kept an hourly record that I realised that I feel a bit better if I have social contact and if I get overtired I feel more hopeless and stuck.'

ASSESSING PROGRESS

Regular measures are a worthwhile investment (but don't overdo things and stress your patient). A series of ratings allows you to obtain a baseline and then to review this against later scores – which will then reveal the impact of interventions. It is particularly important to gather data at the beginning and end of treatment so that overall progress can be assessed.

Using a simple log, a woman with social phobia noted (i) how many social gatherings she attended each week (these were specified), (ii) how many people she spoke to, (iii) how long she stayed. She also completed a Social Phobia Scale at the beginning of her treatment and at monthly intervals there-after. Reviewing her logs and her questionnaire results helped her to see her overall progress (which was motivating), but she also recognised when her results weren't quite as good as she'd hoped, e.g. premenstrually or when she had little time to prepare herself. This helped her better understand her ongoing vulnerabilities and her formulation could be revised accordingly.

GETTING THE MOST FROM THE ASSESSMENTS

Some time ago, two colleagues and I wrote a CBT textbook (Kennerley et al., 2017) and we realised that if you combined our CBT experience, we weren't far short of a hundred years. It amused us and shocked us in equal measure. However, between us we had developed some principles of good practice and here are our suggestions for getting the most from the assessments, our 'top tips'.

Focus on a recent event

Whatever your choice of assessment, a good strategy is to ask your patient to review a recent occasion when they experienced the problem. This makes it easier to access thoughts and feelings. In some cases, it can also be helpful to assess different stages of a problem, e.g. a person's feelings, thoughts and behaviour before, during and after a trauma, or in the build-up to a binge as well as during the binge and in the aftermath.

'I'll only binge if I'm very hungry or stressed, but once I've given myself permission I feel relaxed and excited at the same time. I'll often go on a binge-buy and I'll enjoy shopping for forbidden foods. But when I binge it's quite different. I start to feel numb, and it doesn't take long before I actually don't want to eat any more but I can't stop. And then afterwards I hate myself, I feel wretched and I just want to sleep, cry or vomit (and sometimes I do all three) ...'

This example reminds us that sometimes understanding a problem requires four-dimensional thinking, and this will be reflected in a collection of maintaining cycles in the formulation.

Explain why it will be helpful

Share a meaningful rationale – any of us is more likely to comply if we understand why we need to do something onerous or difficult. Sometimes an initial trial of monitoring might help your patient see the relevance of it. Only continue monitoring as long as it is useful, but bear in mind that it is helpful to have some measures that are continued throughout treatment, such as, mood ratings, so that you can look at variations over the course of treatment.

Keep it relevant

Ensure that there is a good reason for collecting the information. Make the questionnaire meaningful, not just routine; keep your interview questions focused, hypothesis-testing enquiries and not random exploration; check that the attractive template that you've downloaded is actually fit for purpose. Don't gather information for the sake of it.

Keep it simple

Begin with a limited and meaningful task that does not ask too much. As your patient becomes more persuaded of the value of monitoring, and becomes more skilled, you can increase the demands, but still keep in mind the difficulty of observing and recording.

A depressed man began treatment by going out each day for a short walk, and he recorded how long he walked (in minutes) and how much he enjoyed it (on a 10-point scale of enjoyment). This was just about manageable given his depressed state, but as treatment progressed and his mood and motivation improved, he also began to record NATs, to rate how critical his wife was (on a 10-point scale), and to record the three best things he had done that day (a simple list). In addition, he was soon able to monitor specific activities/tasks for particular purposes. He felt it was doable because the tasks had been introduced gradually.

Keep instructions simple – they are easily forgotten or misremembered. It can be helpful to record instructions in a notebook or on a smart phone.

Be specific and clear

Improve the reliability of your measures by spelling out in detail what is to be recorded.

You could refine asking someone to record the frequency with which they 'get anxious in public' by saying, 'People have different experiences of anxiety, what does *get anxious* mean to you. What are we looking out for?'. You then might discover that, for this particular person, it means becoming withdrawn, feeling physically unstable and hot, being snippy with people, getting out of a situation. Now you both know what you are focusing on. Next you could devise a scale to capture how severe this was at any one time.

The advantage of *operationalising* recordings in this way is that, should an incident occur, your patient would easily recognise whether this met the definition of 'get anxious', it would be clear from the agreed criteria.

Use aids to recording

Minimise demand by using frameworks and templates if appropriate, at least in the early stages of therapy. Some can be downloaded from the internet (but do review these with a critical eye) while others can be drawn up with a patient. You can then make copies as required. Record sheets should be as simple and discreet as possible because patients often feel uncomfortable being seen recording personal information.

Give training

Even if the task appears straightforward, always go through a recent example to practise the recording process. This way you will know that the task is clear and you can discuss difficulties that crop up. This way, the patient is tutored in the *skill* of self-monitoring.

Encourage recording as soon as possible after an event

Delayed recall will be less vivid and/or could be biased by mood at the time of completing the record. Sometimes it just isn't possible to record an experience as it happens but encourage patients to complete the task as soon as they can. Alternatively, it may be possible to make a brief note at the time and then complete the full monitoring when it is more convenient.

Review properly

Always look at the information that has been collected   put reviewing it on the agenda. Often, the information is valuable, and the next session often relies on it; but in any case, a patient's efforts should be recognised, so that they will be motivated to continue monitoring in future.

A series of ratings can often be summarised as a simple graph showing change over time. However, a series of *diaries* may be more difficult to summarise because the information is difficult to categorise. So, you might find that asking your patient to review: 'What this is telling me' is a useful way forward, particularly as this targets shifts in cognitions. This exercise also helps patients develop the skill of 'reading' a diary and getting the most out of data collection:

Therapist: Looking over your diaries from the past two weeks, what changes can you see? What have you learnt?

Trish: There's that theme of *get active–feel less depressed* and there is still a pattern of things being worse in the morning. I can see that going out with Hal cheers me – that's why I've been doing that more often.

Th: On our 1–10 scale, how do you feel in the morning? And how do you feel when you are with Hal?

Trish: Between 2–3 in the morning and between 6–8 with Hal. Actually, if you look at my original diary, my rating was 1–2 in the morning and social events were only 4.

Th: What do you make of that?

Trish: Things are getting a bit better and I should keep up my contact with Hal?

Th: Very possibly. How does it feel if you've been active, particularly if you've met up with Hal?

Trish: If I just go for a walk then I get up to a 5 (but it doesn't last very long), if I do some exercise then I get up to a 6 and it lasts longer; if I meet up with Hal I can get 8s and it lasts for a few hours.

Th: So, what might that suggest?

Trish: The more active I am the better I feel, and the best activity is social – especially having contact with Hal.

Th: If we consider everything that you've gleaned from your diary today, there really is *a lot* of useful information there. I wonder if it might be helpful to summarise it. How would you sum up your progress from looking at your diaries?

Trish: It's still very hard: every day is a challenge, but I now know that there are things I can do to shift my mood and the mornings just might be getting easier because of what I'm doing.

Th: When we started therapy you said 'There's no point in trying, I'll never feel better,' and you believed that 90%. How does what you've just said fit with that?

Trish: Recovery is slow, but I am changing my mind: *I am making progress.*

Th: How about writing that down as your summary of the week and giving it a rating?

Trish: Okay – and I'd give it a 60% rating right now (but it might not be so good in the morning).

Here the therapist has used a series of enquiries to help Trish explore the information in the diary and to arrive at an authentic new conclusion about progress – a Socratic approach that we will revisit in Chapter 7.

As the treatment progresses, the responsibility for collating and interpreting information can increasingly be handed over to your patients. You can ask them to review their own diaries and identify themes or the most important incident to discuss. This helps them develop the ability to review and prioritise, which is necessary for effective problem-solving (see Chapter 9).

Live observation

Assessments can go beyond retrospective review and can take place in real-life situations (in vivo) or in role-played activities. This often results in valuable insights that might not emerge from discussion alone.

In vivo

Observing a person at the time the problem occurs can provide information that might otherwise be forgotten or go unnoticed. Sometimes, you can observe behaviour in naturalistic settings:

Laurie and his therapist took a brief walk outside the office and the therapist was able to see the extent to which Laurie averted his gaze in casual social interactions, something that Laurie did not realise.

At other times, you might contrive a situation:

Grace and her therapist went to his office washroom so that the therapist could observe just how Grace washed her hands after touching a washroom door handle. He realised that Grace had not described some of the details of the ritual, including that she washed the soap itself and put it back on the sink after completing each stage in handwashing.

These observations mean that you can judge for yourself the extent of a problem and you can discover important details that may be outside a patient's awareness.

Do consider safety, both for you and the patient. On a home assessment visit, I was once greeted at the door by a patient with a knife in her hand because voices were telling her that I was dangerous. I was relieved that I had asked the patient's community nurse to accompany me because together we were able to calm her and ensure that the situation was safe for us all.

Role play

With the permission of your patient, this approach can be used to recreate a relevant situation in session:

Benji was nervous about asserting himself at work, quite convinced that he spoke unclearly and looked 'odd' when he asked for something for himself. Through role play his therapist was able to observe Benji's interpersonal skills and properly appreciate just how difficult he found the situation. She was also able to give him some useful feedback – namely that he was rather fluent and did not look odd at all in her view. They then agreed to repeat the role play but this time video-recording it so that Benji could see his performance for himself.

The technique of role play is elaborated in Chapter 8 as a Socratic method that uses enactment.

You can, of course, use the full range of measures while observing your patient, including frequency counts and rating scales. So, Grace could have rated her anxiety before, during and/ or after washing.

Other informants

Although most of the information used in adult services therapy is provided by the patient, other informants (a partner or best friend, for example) can augment this. Consider interviewing others (or collecting written information from them) because:

- *they may have information unavailable to your patient* – for example, a man may believe he behaves oddly in social situations, and someone else's view could confirm or contradict; a partner may report that your patient is very quiet and initiates little conversation whether at home or out socially, and this may not be obvious to that patient;
- *the problem may impact on another person and exacerbate it* – for example, a patient with obsessional problems may involve relatives or other significant people in their rituals,

thereby stressing them; this in turn creates an environmental tension that can worsen the obsessional problem;

- *the way someone else responds to the patient's problems may help maintain it* – for example, reassurance-giving or being overly critical are common examples of interpersonal maintenance of a problem;
- *a significant other's beliefs about a problem might influence the beliefs of your patient* – for example, that medication is likely to be the only effective solution; that the patient is a bad person; that avoidance is always the best solution.

Informants can be approached in a similar way to patients, recognising that they will need to be engaged and possibly educated about CBT. Issues of confidentiality also need to be discussed with both the patient and informants, to establish what might be disclosed and how risk is managed.

Watch out for …

Assessment doesn't always go smoothly – but remember that you can always use a setback as a learning opportunity (look back over what we have been saying about Relapse Management). Typical stumbling blocks include the following:

Struggles with literacy

Data-collecting is simply a means to an end so consider other modalities for recording relevant data, e.g. speaking into a mobile phone, using symbols rather than written words. Always ask your patient for advice – they often have the best ideas because they've probably tackled similar obstacles.

Patient observations have therapeutic effects

Active data collection can have pro- or anti-therapeutic effects. These findings can add to the understanding of a patient's strengths and needs, and therefore add to your formulation with conclusions such as 'If I stand back and consider my problem I can manage it,' or 'If I focus on my problem it becomes worse.'

Once I started to keep a record of what I was eating I found that I was cutting back. I hadn't realised how much I snacked between meals and each time I was about to snack I noted it, and this meant that I paused for thought and decided not to eat between meals.

When I tried to keep track of my self-doubting thoughts, I was so aware that I needed to note them I couldn't keep them out of my mind.

Anxiety levels are static (or worsening) as a patient makes behavioural progress

This is usually because a person is doing more, taking more risks, pushing despite the anxiety. The lack of improvement in scores can be demoralising, so do discuss it and make sure that you have a way of capturing and recognising behavioural achievements.

Overuse of questionnaires can lead to a familiarity that undermines accuracy

Dan completed the PHQ-9 before every session. He became so familiar with the items that he stopped really reading each question and became careless in completing the questionnaire. If he felt that things were relatively OK, he would simply check all the 'Not at all' responses, and if things were pretty difficult for him, he'd check all the 'Nearly every day' responses. This was less taxing for him but it meant that he and his therapist lost sight of subtle fluctuations in his mood.

Some standardised measures have parallel forms that you can use to avoid this problem but most of the assessments we use in CBT don't. Again, it is clear that you need to review responses with your patient to establish how true they are, but you also could ask yourself if you really need to collect such detailed information so frequently. In Dan's case it might have been more useful to administer the questionnaire only at the beginning of treatment, at review sessions and on discharge. If you want to keep a closer eye on session-to-session changes then you might negotiate a simple rating of wellbeing – perhaps a five-point scale – to be completed at the start of each meeting.

SUMMARY

- Assessment and formulation work hand in hand, and patient and therapist work together to develop the optimum means of gathering relevant data.
- There are many ways to collect relevant information and you need to consider your choices carefully so that they are reliable, valid, timely and user-friendly.
- You need to use assessment throughout the course of therapy – but do not overuse assessments.
- Much information will come from your patient but your observations or the observations of key others can contribute.
- Observations can be live or retrospective.

REFLECTION & ACTION

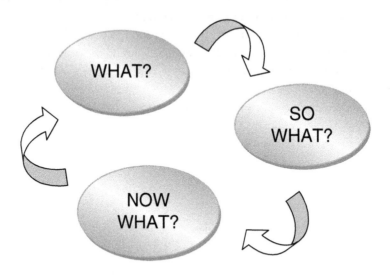

WHAT are you taking away from this chapter? What teaching points resonate with you?

....
....
....
....
....
....
....
....
....

SO WHAT? What significance do these points have – how do they relate to your previous learning or views? Do they challenge your former opinions? Have you gleaned new ideas for helping patients or indeed looking after your own needs?

....

....

....

....

....

....

....

....

....

....

NOW WHAT? How will you now approach your assessments? What are you now going to do differently? Make a commitment with yourself to follow through on at least one of your new ideas.

....

....

....

....

....

....

....

....

....

....

7

SOCRATIC METHODS: ENQUIRY, REFLECTION AND LOGS

In 1993, in a large lecture theatre in London, Dr Christine Padesky held the audience's attention as she spoke about Socratic methods in CBT. She recognised their versatility, calling them 'the cornerstone of cognitive therapy', but crucially she reminded us that Socratic methods are about *guiding discovery* not *changing minds*. In using Socratic methods in CBT we aim to ask not to tell.

Why? Because CBT therapists are at times trainers and coaches, helping people learn new possibilities and new ways of being, and it is well established that we learn better if we draw our own conclusions rather than if we are simply told the answer (Barrett, Crucian, Schwarz & Heilman, 2000; Erdelyi, Buschke & Finkelstein, 1977). Socrates possibly appreciated this when he developed his method of encouraging students to evolve their own deductions. Beck knew this when he advised 'Cognitive therapy uses primarily the Socratic method' (Beck et al. 1985: 177).

Effective Socratic methods have three key characteristics:

1. *They are hypothesis driven.* As therapists we have a hunch that we check out. Questions and exercises shouldn't be used randomly or just because they are in the protocol. What we do should be justified by our hypotheses concerning problem origin, maintenance or recovery.
2. *Questions are answerable.* They enable a person to realise something for themselves, using a personal knowledge base to form new opinions and see new possibilities.
3. *The new perspective enlightens* a person in some way, enabling them to revise old conclusions and/or see new ways forward. We want an 'ah ha' rather than a 'so what?' response.

I once saw a therapist ask a very demoralised patient 'So your mother was an expert in child psychology?' The hypothesis was that the patient wholly believed his mother's harsh criticism of him as a youngster because he overestimated her understanding of child development and needs. The response was dramatic. The patient's face broke into a huge smile as he replied 'No. No, she knew nothing about raising kids or what they needed,' and with this he realised that his mother's criticisms were founded on ignorance. The simple question had put his experience in perspective and shifted his beliefs and mood state.

But that very same question would have failed if the patient hadn't the personal knowledge to answer it. And it would have failed if the patient's 'no' was simply stating a known fact that didn't impact on his perspective (a 'so what' response) or if the patient had been upset by the question. There are no universally 'good' Socratic questions or exercises – they are posed in a context of hypothesising and sensitive planning.

Socratic methods can be used at all stages of CBT and they embrace a range of interventions including curious enquiry, reflecting dilemmas, reviewing logs, and active experimentation. In this chapter, we will look at the use of Socratic methods that have a verbal emphasis (enquiry, reflection, logs) and those that have an experiential emphasis (behavioural experiments and role play) will be described in Chapter 8. However, the distinction is perhaps misleading as this is *CBT* so the cognitive and the behavioural elements will always go hand in hand.

STAGES IN SOCRATIC METHOD

A common misconception is that Socratic method is all about asking questions, but Socratic *method* is an elegant interweaving of collaborative hypothesis testing, exploration and decision-making that results in guided discovery. During this process, patients should not feel interrogated but engaged in a genuinely curious conversation. It is a conversation that is carefully orchestrated by the therapist so that is hypothesis led and patients have the time to reflect and explore.

Padesky's four steps of Socratic Dialogue

In 1993, Padesky described four key steps in the back and forth process of Socratic dialogue (SD) and this nicely captures the verbal aspect of Socratic method:

1. *Asking informational questions*: this generates information about the patient's situation and experiences. This might be factual information ('How many children live at home?') or might reveal meanings ('How do you feel about this?', 'What does that say about you?').

2. *Empathic listening*: essential compassionate listening when the therapist tunes into the patient's experiences, adopts patient language, begins to hypothesise about the patient's problems (in the light of known theory and research) and – importantly – notices what is not said and attends to non-verbal cues.

Steps 1 and 2 work well in tandem as the therapist gathers information, refines hypotheses and checks out those hunches before moving on to step 3 and later step 4:

3. *Summaries*: brief feedback or reflections to summarise and clarify what might be a great deal of information. This also offers an opportunity for collaboration. Summaries can be spoken and/or written and might be followed by returning to step 1 or moving forward to step 4.
4. *Analytical/synthesising questions*: these prompt consolidation and planning. Synthesising questions promote deeper understandings ('How might these ideas fit together?', 'Are there themes here?', 'What have you learnt from this?') while analytical questions encourage taking things forward ('… and given that, what could you do?', 'How could you check that out?').

While SD is largely a verbal process, it is also used to unpack learning from more active investigations (behavioural experiments, thought records, role plays and imagery exercises) and again we are reminded that this is part of a larger *method* of working in CBT. In the next chapter we look at the integration of more behavioural strategies.

Butler's Mind the Gap

Although this chapter is headed 'Socratic Methods', we also consider the role of direct questions and didactic teaching because optimum use of Socratic methods is achieved by balancing direct or didactic with Socratic approaches. As my colleague Gillian Butler pointed out during one of our teaching sessions, one possible outcome of using Socratic technique is that we discover gaps in patients' knowledge and this prompts us to fill those gaps – often didactically.

Art feared shaking in public, so he avoided signing documents or carrying things in front of others. His therapist hypothesised that Art's anxiety caused physical tension and that caused shaking. Hoping to help him make this connection, she asked 'What usually happens in our bodies when we get anxious?'

His reply was 'I don't know. Why are you asking me – what's that got to do with anything?'

Art was unaware of the anxiety/muscle tension/shaking link that seemed obvious to his therapist. She needed to fill this gap in his knowledge. She did this didactically by telling him about the connections, but she could have directed him to reading matter or illustrated the connection by demonstrating her own hand tremor when she overtensed her hand muscles. Once Art had the information, she returned to the Socratic mode by enquiring what he made of this, how it fitted with his experience etc.

Some psychoeducation is best achieved experientially, e.g. teaching assertiveness skills or breathing techniques, and this can combine didactic and Socratic methods. For example, a therapist might model being assertive, and the patient would observe (didactic) whilst being involved in the exercise. The therapist would then prompt them to draw their own conclusions from the experience (Socratic) and to try this out for themselves and reflect on what they had learned (Socratic).

Sometimes the gap will be in the therapist's knowledge. We realise that we need concrete information so we shift to direct questions: 'How long have you been doing this job?'; 'Are you able to retake the exams?'; 'How many children do you have?'. This enables us to refine our hypotheses and then we can test them Socratically:

Therapist: So what is your main difficulty at present? (Direct, information-gathering question)

Patient: My mood, I'm so depressed. I can't shake it off and I can't see it ever getting better.

Th: When did this start to be a problem for you? (Direct, information-gathering question because the therapist needs more information to shape up their hypothesis)

P: It's always been a problem – at least since I was a teenager, but I just got on with it. Since I retired, I've not been able to get rid of this heavy misery.

Th: [Hypothesis: marked to severe depression, worsened by the life event of retirement] Can I ask you a little more about your mood? (Direct question, setting the scene for further exploration and giving the message that the patient has choices thus encouraging them to be more open to Socratic enquiry)

P: OK.

Th: What else goes through your mind when you are low? (A Socratic question to build an understanding of the patient's inner world)

P: That there is no point in carrying on … [falls silent]

Th: [Hypothesis: marked to severe depression, suicidal] Can you say more? (Direct question to discover if the patient is able to elaborate, and also to convey to them that they aren't under pressure to do more than they can tolerate)

P: Well I might as well be dead.

Th: I'm beginning to understand just how bad you must be feeling and I'm sorry to hear that you are so distressed. How often do you feel so low that you believe that you might as well be dead? (Direct question to assess risk)

P: Pretty much all the time.

Th: [Hypothesis: marked to severe depression, suicidal, at risk] I see. Have you made plans? [This begins a series of direct questions to establish risk] … Have you ever made an attempt on your life? … Do you live with someone or alone? etc.

In this example the therapist has helped a patient reveal suicidal thoughts through sensitive balancing of direct and Socratic questions, and then asked focused and direct questions to ascertain risk.

ENQUIRY, REFLECTION AND LOGS

Enquiry

The skill of Socratic enquiry is one that might come more naturally if we do not try too hard. Socratic enquiry helps a person review relevant evidence as widely as possible. We are more likely to obtain this 'bigger picture' by maintaining curiosity and not being too constrained by our own expectations and beliefs; and by frequently asking 'and is there anything else?' If we get bound by rigid expectations, then we might terminate our enquiry before a wide enough data base has been uncovered.

Asking a question is a commonly used Socratic strategy, and of course a cognitive therapist uses many types of question (see James, Morse & Howarth, 2009 for a review). We ask direct, information-gathering questions, ranging from a simple 'What is your address?' to a far more challenging 'Have you made plans to kill yourself?' At other times we ask social questions to put our patients at ease ('How was the trip to Wales at the weekend?', 'Did your son's exams go well?') or we make enquiries to clarify confusion ('Just what was it that she said to you?'). We are not (and should not be) limited to using Socratic questions.

Virtually any enquiry can be Socratic if it conforms to the three criteria above and the questions need not be elaborate. Very simple enquiries such as 'Because?' or 'And then?' can yield much relevant information if timed and communicated well.

A crucial 'tip' from Beck himself is that whatever type of enquiry we choose, we need to give the patient space and time to reflect: 'Questions must be carefully timed and phrased so as to help the patient recognize and consider his notions reflectively – to weigh his thoughts with objectivity,' and a patient 'may feel he is being cross-examined or that he is being attacked if questions are used to "trap" him into contradicting himself' (Beck et al., 1979: 71).

This reminds us that, within CBT, Socratic enquiry is not used to prove the questioner's point – the intention is to encourage patients to rethink their view and then develop new outlooks *when appropriate*. On occasion our explorations will indicate that a patient's upsetting view is accurate, or partially accurate, and then we would help them problem-solve (see Chapter 9):

Therapist: (Hypothesis: the patient is overestimating health threat and does not have cancer: this is based on the patient having had several tests for cancer, all of which have proved negative) And when you visited the doctor to get the test results, what did you learn?

Patient: I didn't have cancer, but they found something called an abdominal aortic aneurysm.

The therapist had been correct in hypothesising that the patient did not have cancer, but now the therapist developed a new hypothesis that reflected the new reality of an actual health threat: 'My patient needs help in dealing with this.' They asked the patient how he felt about the diagnosis, what it meant to him, how he saw the future, and what help he might need from therapy. The patient was able to share that he felt scared and needed help in keeping things in perspective (it was a small aneurysm) so that he could follow the advice of his doctor to lose weight and start taking exercise. The therapist was able to help the patient refine his problem-solving skills so that he could properly attend to his condition while also learning to counter catastrophic thoughts about the aneurysm. The therapist was also aware of the need to keep the patient motivated to change their lifestyle.

Some years ago, Dr Stirling Moorey developed CBT for helping patients in adversity (2002) and his writings remain an excellent resource for guiding therapists working with patients who do have tangible problems.

Using metaphors

Metaphor and analogy can aid Socratic enquiry by encouraging patients to imagine a parallel situation so that their perspective is temporarily shifted from the original view. This typically involves mental shifts in person or in time, elicited by questions such as:

- If you were advising your best friend, what might you say?
- How might your dad, who seems quite upbeat, respond to such a dilemma?
- If your friend were to respond to your concern, what do you think they would say?
- In that situation, what might your son do?
- How might a detective/teacher start to address this?
- When you shift into 'work mode' how would you tackle this?
- When you faced a similar difficulty in your first marriage – how did you resolve it?
- What would the younger you, before you had this problem, be thinking or doing?
- If you fast forwarded a couple of years and this was no longer a problem, how do you imagine you might view yourself?

In considering such possibilities, a person not only decentres but also enters a different mind-set and this is likely to trigger different emotions (less negative). Thus, the strong emotion of the personal situation is tempered, and your patient may be able to think more productively.

A number of techniques involve very systematic enquiry such that the process is a recognisable stand-alone strategy. Four very useful such interventions are: 'Downward arrowing', 'Responsibility Pie', the 'Continuum technique', and Butler's 'Decision-making tree'.

Downward arrowing

There is a particular type of enquiry that aims to systematically elaborate on, or 'unpack', a person's experience or ATs and perhaps identify the more fundamental meanings underlying an unwanted reaction. In some texts it is called 'vertical arrow restructuring', but it is most commonly referred to as 'downward arrowing'.

If you use the downward arrow technique, your questions should be paced and phrased so that your patient never feels interrogated, but rather that you are taking a genuine interest. You might begin a line of enquiry with enquiries like:

- 'I wonder, just how did you feel at the time?'
- '… and what was going through your mind?'
- 'Any particular thoughts or pictures?'
- 'That's interesting – could you say a bit more?'
- 'That sounds really relevant – could you expand on just how you felt? What you thought?'

These types of question reactivate the affect of the moment and focus on relevant cognitions.

Babs avoided leaving the house. She was not immediately able to explain this other than saying that being out in public 'felt bad' even if she was only a few metres from home. When asked some of the questions above, she was able to explain that she felt 'uncomfortable', that she felt 'awkward', and eventually she said that she felt ' … as though people are looking at me' – in fact she had a fleeting image of this.

This initial line of enquiry might be followed by further enquiry to gently tease out the personal relevance of a thought or an image – questions such as:

- 'I wonder what seems so bad about that?'
- 'In your view, what does that mean?'
- 'What does that say about you?'
- 'What would that mean about your life/your future?'
- 'What do you imagine others would think of you?'
- 'How would you label that?'
- 'Can you describe the worst thing that could happen?'
- '… and if that were true – then what?'

This way, you and your patient can discover more about the belief system relating to a particular problem.

Babs was able to state that she believed that people were critical of her, that they thought she was 'bubble gum'. Saying this reduced her to tears. When asked what 'bubble gum' meant to her she said that it was dreadful because it confirmed her own belief that she was worthless, stupid, something that people spat out and walked away from, forgettable.

Interestingly, the words 'worthless, stupid, forgettable … ' did not provoke the strong emotion that was triggered by 'bubble gum.' This is a reminder of the importance of uncovering the idiosyncratic image, word or phrase that holds the patient's distress.

Like many patients, Babs found downward arrowing emotionally-charged. For this reason, it should be used thoughtfully, only if we can justify it, and with permission:

- 'Is it alright for me to continue with these questions?'
- 'Do you need a bit of a break? Let me know if you do.'

Even then we need to pace this sensitively, accept periods of silence, look for ways of making the task easier, and we must be ready to stop the exploration if someone finds it too distressing. Once the relevant cognitions have been identified, they can be examined and tested using cognitive testing (see the next section) and behavioural experiment (see Chapter 8).

It is worth remembering that during this exercise you can also discover functional, positive beliefs, such as 'On the whole, people seem to like me,' or 'If I put in the effort, I can get things done.' Sometimes more positive beliefs are simply revealed as part of the course of enquiry, but we can increase the likelihood of uncovering these if we ask questions such as 'What would be so good about that? How might that help you? What positive things does that suggest?' Such beliefs can enhance progress (e.g. someone who believes himself likeable and capable is likely to engage well with you, can probably take on quite challenging social assignments and would be motivated to engage in homework tasks) so it is useful to identify them. They can also contribute to the positive aspects of formulations (see Chapter 4).

Through downward arrowing, the patient's fundamental belief system is often revealed (as in Babs's case). This is sometimes referred to as 'the bottom line' (Fennell, 1999), although it is often more akin to a 'bottom triangle', comprising the elements of Beck et al.'s (1979) cognitive triad: beliefs about the self, others and the world, and the future. These elements relate to each other, and finding yourself going around the triangle is often an indication that the 'bottom' has been reached:

Babs revealed that she believed that she was stupid (self). She then said that this left her feeling socially different (others), isolated and she predicted lonely years ahead (future). That image of loneliness then strengthened her conviction that she was stupid and different.

It can take several sessions before the core belief system is revealed, and sometimes it is simply not accessible. In fact, it is not always necessary to reach the bottom line (or triangle) in order to carry out effective CBT, and much productive work can be, and should be, carried out at the level of an AT or with the rules and assumptions associated with core beliefs. This is how Beck and his colleagues envisaged CBT working (1979). However, there can be advantages in uncovering core beliefs not least because an awareness of them can help us understand persistent vulnerabilities: '*It's no wonder that I have no social confidence and am depressed if I feel so bad and undesirable.*'

There is always a danger that if you have a strong belief in a hypothesis you may use the downward arrow technique simply to pursue its confirmation (to 'change minds'). Do remember that however well-informed we might be, we are sometimes wrong. A great strength of Socratic dialogue, provided that it is coupled with curiosity and humility, is that it can lead us to conclusions that we did not anticipate. A useful rule when using the technique is to devise questions that might *refute* your hypothesis. When you think that you have confirmed your hunch, ask another question or two designed to disprove your theory. This both helps you refute an incorrect hypothesis and also guards against your being too narrow in focus.

Responsibility Pie

Greenberger and Padesky (2016) describe this technique succinctly and clearly in their book *Mind over mood*. They developed the Responsibility Pie strategy to help people to weigh personal responsibility fairly. It comprises four clear steps:

Step 1: Rate responsibility for an action or event (X).
Step 2: List all those persons and aspects of a situation that contributed to X. Own name is added to the end of the list.
Step 3: Draw a circle to represent a 'pie' and apportion 'slices' of responsibility for each name on the list, based on percentage ratings for each. Sometimes this step is redundant (see the example) as the new conclusion can be drawn from Step 2.
Step 4: Drawing a new conclusion from either Step 2 or Step 3 and rerating responsibility.

Hester believed that she was 95% responsible for her son's hyperactive behaviours in the infant school. This fitted with her long-standing view of herself as flawed and incompetent. Her therapist asked her to brainstorm anyone else, or anything else, that might also carry some responsibility. It was a challenging task because Hester was so used to blaming herself, but with encouragement she came up with the following:

- The school staff who should be able to help Paulie learn how to manage activity outbursts.
- The fact that the school is understaffed so it is difficult to give Paulie extra attention.
- The kids who share foods with additives even though I ask Paulie not to take them.
- The child who always seems to wind up Paulie by calling him 'Pee-pee'.
- The ADHD that has recently been diagnosed.
- The routine at school that no longer allows Paulie to have an afternoon nap.
- Paulie – he has an exuberant character.
- Me.

At this stage Hester looked at the list and her expression changed. Her therapist asked the synthesising question 'What do you make of this?' and Hester said that a penny had dropped. She could see that she was only one of many players in this problem, and when asked to now rate her responsibility she estimated 25% at most. Her therapist then asked 'And how does that leave you feeling?' to which she replied that she felt liberated, not so worthless – but she also appreciated that she did carry a significant amount of responsibility as Paulie's mother and she asked her therapist to help her be more assertive with the school so that she could better argue on his behalf.

Had she drawn a 'Pie' it would have looked like this:

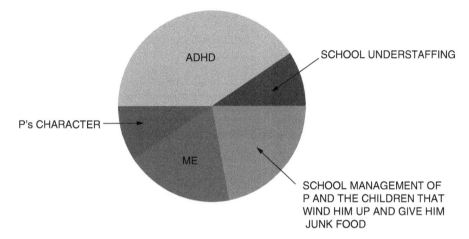

Figure 7.1   Responsibility Pie

The continuum technique

Padesky (1994) has described this as an essential schema-change strategy, but it is so versatile that it can be regarded as an invaluable technique for helping any patient combat dichotomous thinking and develop the skill of discrimination. The continuum technique, sometimes referred to as 'scaling' (Pretzer, 1990), is relevant when 'all or nothing' thinking (see Chapter 1) underpins the problem.

From time to time you might well pick up on an inner construct of opposites, where the dichotomy is usually negative–positive; very good–very bad; heroes–villains ... you get the picture (see Table 7.1). You might also discover that your patient will place themselves in the negative category and only consider leaving that 'box' if their achievement or experience is extreme: 100% success in something, for example.

Quite predictably, extreme thinking drives extreme emotions and these in turn can drive extreme behaviours. For example, a person who believes they are a total failure might feel deeply despondent and so give up on task – which will support the belief that they are a failure. The trap closes. What we need to do is help them appreciate the gradations between

Failure and *Success*. Padesky urges us to establish continua that run from a neutral position to a positive position, and if this is possible it might be beneficial to underplay the negative, but sometimes a continuum without the negative dimension does not have credibility, and so you will need to check your patient's view of this.

Table 7.1 Dichotomous thinking

Extreme negative	Extreme positive
[I'm a] total failure	Success in everything
[I] can't trust anyone	Trust everyone
[I'm] unlovable	Always 100% lovable
The worst will happen [to me]	I have good fortune always

Jo struggled to control her eating – she regularly binged and then vomited. The trigger for this was twofold: (i) an extreme view of eating (that semi-starvation was 'success' and eating more than 1000 calories or eating starchy foods was 'failure'); (ii) an extreme view of performance, namely that success was only achieved if performance was outstanding. When Jo perceived herself either failing on the eating or the performance front, she tended to write herself off and turn to comfort bingeing.

In therapy she was asked if she could imagine her own behaviour (work performance or eating) falling between the two extremes. She said no. When she and her therapist explored Jo's perspective, she could only see less than perfect was the same as failure.

So, her therapist asked her to imagine a friend and consider if there were behaviours that fell between the extremes. Jo could do this for a friend (and hence realised that she held higher standards for herself than for others) and with some Socratic enquiry from her therapist developed two hierarchies – one for work performance and one for eating. She then populated the spectrum between two extremes.

The criteria for each continuum were refined to minimise ambiguity (e.g. clarifying what Jo meant by 'average' and by 'junk food') and then these two continua served as a reference that helped Jo re-evaluate her own performance.

It felt uncomfortable at first, but Jo became adept at calibrating her behaviour. Her therapist could then review (Socratically) what Jo had learned from this – she said that she had discovered that it was safe to be less than perfect and if she was more lenient with herself, her mood was more moderate and she binged less.

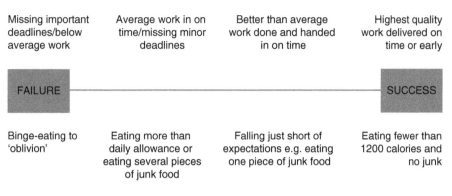

Missing important deadlines/below average work

Average work in on time/missing minor deadlines

Better than average work done and handed in on time

Highest quality work delivered on time or early

FAILURE ———————————————————— SUCCESS

Binge-eating to 'oblivion'

Eating more than daily allowance or eating several pieces of junk food

Falling just short of expectations e.g. eating one piece of junk food

Eating fewer than 1200 calories and no junk

Figure 7.2 Jo's continua for work and eating

Devising continua often leads on to behavioural experiments, such as practising handing in work that falls short of perfect or eating a single piece of junk food, but BEs are explored in the next chapter.

Decision-making tree

Worry ('What if … ?') and rumination ('If only … ') often lock people into unproductive cycles of negative thinking and increasing distress. After years of researching worry, Dr Gillian Butler wisely concluded that it's not worth worrying about the things you *can* do something about and it's not worth worrying about the things that you *can't* do something about. A simple concept but not always easy to enact. To help people make the most of her view she developed a decision-making framework (based on decentring, distraction and problem-solving) that can help manage both worries and ruminations (Butler, Grey & Hope, 2018).

Her decision-making tree is summarised in Figure 7.3. It starts with a clear statement of concern because none of us can address vague notions. We need to be specific: e.g. 'What if I'm unwell?' is a worry but it needs to be transformed from a question to a statement; 'I am concerned about my health,' is better, but still rather vague; 'I am worried that I have breast cancer,' is specific and more easily addressed.

Once the concern is specific the next step is deciding if anything can be done. If it can, then a plan can be made and executed; if not, then distraction comes into play. And this can be done over and over.

In this way there is always something that a person can do that prevents them getting stuck in a worry or rumination loop – and the solutions are self-generated, which makes this an elegant Socratic tool.

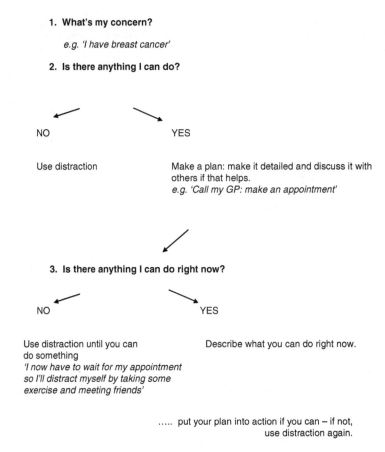

1. **What's my concern?**

   e.g. 'I have breast cancer'

2. **Is there anything I can do?**

NO

YES

Use distraction

Make a plan: make it detailed and discuss it with others if that helps.
e.g. 'Call my GP: make an appointment'

3. **Is there anything I can do right now?**

NO

YES

Use distraction until you can do something
'I now have to wait for my appointment so I'll distract myself by taking some exercise and meeting friends'

Describe what you can do right now.

….. put your plan into action if you can – if not, use distraction again.

Figure 7.3   Decision-making tree

Reflection

The previous strategies have relied heavily on Socratic enquiry, posing questions to help patients develop new ideas. However, we can use more than questions to direct attention towards possibilities previously outside awareness.

For example, we can *reflect dilemmas* to prompt a new perspective:

Therapist: It sounds as though you really want to stop cutting yourself but equally you really feel you need the relief it gives you.

Patient: I hadn't thought of it that way – no wonder I feel trapped and frustrated.

We can simply *summarise*:

Therapist: Let me see if I can sum up, then. If you don't do as your sister asks, she calls you lazy and if you do she criticises your performance?

Patient: That sounds rather harsh, but I suppose if I'm honest that is how it is. I can see now that I'm never going to be okay in her eyes and that's probably why I feel the way I do.

We can offer information:

Therapist: When any of us feels threatened the brain prepares us for flight, fight or freeze: it's how we've evolved. What do you make of that?

Patient: That it's not my fault that I freeze – I am not simply weak.

Capsule summaries often provide excellent opportunities for reflection so don't forget to make the most of these, too.

Logs that focus on cognitions or emotions

We commonly ask our patients to keep records and diaries, some very simple and others comprehensive. Whatever the structure these logs can be a medium for discovery simply by asking questions such as 'So what do you make of that entry, just there?', 'What did you discover from keeping a note of this over the week?', 'Did anything strike you as a recurring theme?', 'Did you notice any patterns?'.

A five-column thought record is possibly the most widely used of the CBT logs. It is a sophisticated Socratic tool because it prompts the user to observe, review and reformulate so new perspectives are self-generated. Over time this evolves into an automatic skill enabling a person to stand back and review NATs effectively.

The original format for a thought record can be found in Beck's 1979 manual, but it has been modified over time to give additional opportunity to consider why it is understandable that a NAT might cross one's mind (this encourages a compassionate attitude) and what might not support that NAT, before moving on to considering what might be a rational response to a particular situation.

A typical record can be seen in Figure 7.4 (Automatic thought record).

These records need to be negotiated with patients so you can be sure that they have credibility and are manageable. They can be made bespoke by using a patient's vocabulary and the columns can be introduced gradually so as not to overwhelm them. It is quite usual to complete only the first four columns to begin with. Then, as patients become more adept at self-monitoring, you can introduce the remaining columns.

You should always trial a thought diary by taking a patient through each step, using their own experiences. The questions that we typically use when we engage in a cognitive review can enhance the exploration of compassionate understandings and new possibilities, and help patients engage with the thought record and build a repertoire of questions they can pose for themselves at a later stage. Typical phrases might include:

- 'So how did that leave you feeling?'
- 'And what was running through your mind at the time?'
- 'Thoughts? Images?'
- 'In your experience, what fits with this thought, what makes it seem true?'
- 'Why might any of us have that thought at some time?'
- 'I'm just wondering, do you have any experience of this not being the case?'
- 'Is there anything that doesn't seem to fit with that thought?'
- 'How might someone else view the situation?'
- 'Is that so all of the time, or are there occasions when things are different?'
- 'Before you were depressed, what would have gone through your mind at that point?'
- 'If you were responding to your best friend, what would you say?'
- 'Now that you have looked at the bigger picture, how would you view your original concern?'
- 'Given what you've just described, how likely do you think it is that the worst will happen?'
- 'If you reflect on what we've discussed what picture comes to mind now?', 'And what message does that carry for you?'
- 'How helpful, or unhelpful, is it to hold this particular belief?'
- 'I'm curious, what good, if any, comes of holding this belief?'
- 'What could be the downside of seeing things this way?'
- 'If you see the world this way, how do you feel, how do others react?'

Another widely-used log is the Positive data log (Padesky, 1994). This encourages patients to selectively attend to accomplishments, achievements, compliments, strengths etc. The idea is that patients build a persuasive log of worth while developing the skill of appreciating the positive in themselves.

An excellent guide to this can be found in Melanie Fennell's (2016) book *Overcoming low self-esteem.*

Figure 7.4 Automatic thought record

Automatic Thought Record

Monitor your feelings and beliefs by rating them using the following scale:

Absent		Moderate		Strong	
0	1 2 3	4 5 6	7 8		

Date Time	EMOTION Rate Emotion 0–8	SITUATION What triggered the problem emotion?	AUTOMATIC THOUGHT/ IMAGE (COGNITION) Rate belief in this 0–8	IT'S UNDERSTANDABLE THAT I SEE THINGS THIS WAY BECAUSE …	HOWEVER … What doesn't fit with this view?	NEW CONCLUSION Rating my belief in this new conclusion 0–8	EMOTION Re-rate Emotion 0–8
Wed 10am	Sad: 6/8	Day off work. Lying in bed.	What's the point? Things are grim and won't get better. 7/8	My mood is low and many things have gone badly recently – despite my best efforts.	However, some things have gone well. I got a tax refund that I wasn't expecting. I forced myself to go out with J and it was a good evening.	I'm low. I'm ruminating and I'm forgetting the good things. It's not brilliant right now but it's not completely awful. There are things that I can do to make a difference. 6/8	Sad: 3/8

(Continues)

Figure 7.4 (Continued)

Date Time	EMOTION Rate Emotion 0–8	SITUATION What triggered the problem emotion?	AUTOMATIC THOUGHT/ IMAGE (COGNITION) Rate belief in this 0–8	IT'S UNDERSTANDABLE THAT I SEE THINGS THIS WAY BECAUSE …	HOWEVER … What doesn't fit with this view?	NEW CONCLUSION Rating my belief in this new conclusion 0–8	EMOTION Re-rate Emotion 0–8
Sat noon	Scared: 7/8	Asked to drive to the other office with a package. I can't tell the boss I'm scared.	I'm not fit to drive. I'll have an accident. I'm useless. 8/8	My concentration is poor right now and I'm a nervous driver at the best of times so I think that I could have an accident on the motorway section. It's a company car and I'm not used to it.	I did some driving last weekend (not motorway). I've used company cars in the past and they are automatic so that should help. Also – my concentration was not bad this morning.	This won't be easy but I think that I can do it if I relax myself before I set off and keep my wits about me. I can take my time – no rush – and I can by-pass the motorway section if necessary. 7/8	Scared: 4/8
Sun 11am	Sad: 6/8 Afraid: 6/8	Day off work (again). Lying in bed (again).	I don't want to feel like this. I'm scared I'm going to go under again. 7/8	I did drink a lot last night and I never feel good the next day. I can feel my mood slipping and I've had some really bad depressions so I am scared that I'm going to that black place again.	I functioned quite well at work on Thursday thru' Saturday and I did have some moments of feeling ok and enjoying parts of my job.	Lying in bed (especially with a hangover) makes me feel worse. I am at a stage of good days and bad days and this will possibly turn into a good day if I find something to do. 6/8	Sad: 2/8 Afraid: 3/8

Lola knew that she had long-standing low self-esteem (LSE) and she wanted to address this. Her therapist asked her to imagine a friend who did not suffer from LSE, and then asked Lola to say what she saw in her friend that revealed her good self-esteem. Lola very quickly listed: ' … she accepts compliments, she gives herself credit for completing tasks at work, when someone says thank you she accepts this, she treats herself to nice things and simply enjoys it.' Next her therapist asked Lola to think of a word or a phrase that summed up the attitude of a person like her friend, and Lola replied 'It's as if she believes "I matter".' Now they had the basis for a positive data log to help Lola enhance her self-esteem.

At the beginning of the exercise the therapist asked Lola how much she believed that she mattered and she replied 2/8. This was their baseline. Next, they used the criteria that Lola had generated as a reminder of the sort of things that she could do in order to gather data to support the possibility that she mattered:

- Accepting compliments (saying 'thank you' rather than dismissing them).
- Giving myself credit for achievements (if I would give a friend credit, I must give myself credit – this includes work and social achievements).
- Treating myself and giving myself permission to do pleasurable things for myself.

Her first few days of using the log are summarised in Figure 7.5.

In order to have full impact it helps if these logs go beyond simple data-collecting. Entries in the final column ('What this tells me') and the final row ('What I have learnt') invite the patient to be Socratic in reviewing their learning.

WHEN NOT TO OPT FOR SOCRATIC METHODS

At the risk of repetition, an effective clinician is one who gets the right balance between Socratic and non-Socratic methods. There are occasions when a direct question or a didactic approach will better progress therapy, for example:

- *Mind the gap*: when your patient does not have the basic knowledge to benefit from Socratic methods.
- *Risk*: when you need swift and unambiguous information.
- *Information gathering*: when nothing is to be gained by using a Socratic approach, be direct.

There are other times when it is wise to ponder when a Socratic approach risks colluding with avoidance, or encouraging worry and rumination, or reflects reassurance giving.

Figure 7.5 Positive data log

Positive Data Log: *gathering evidence that 'I matter'*

When you notice one of the following, make a note of it before you forget:

- Someone paid me a compliment
- I completed a work task on time
- I did something just for me
- I did a kindness for others
- Someone said 'thank you'

	Absent	Moderate	Strong
	0 1 2 3	4 5 6	7 8

Date/Time	WHAT HAPPENED	WHAT THIS TELLS ME How much I believe this 0–8
Wed afternoon	I completed a report early and my line manager had reviewed it by lunch time. He said that it was a fluent and concise piece of writing that would be very helpful in the upcoming departmental review.	I can do good work that benefits others – therefore what I do matters. 6/8 My boss is impressed by my work. He probably/possibly thinks I matter. 4/8
Thurs evening	I was exhausted so I forced myself to relax. I did what my friend would have done: bubble bath, candles and then watched a good film in bed. It felt unusual to be so nice to myself, but it felt good.	I feel better and sleep better if I look after myself. 8/8 It's ok to indulge myself. 8/8 I matter enough to spoil myself. 3/8
Sat noon	Met up with Gerry – who has been quite low – for lunch and we laughed a lot. She thanked me for a great time and wants to do this again.	I made a difference in Gerry's life. I matter to her. 5/8 I can take thanks and feel ok about it. 7/8
Sun morning	Got up early to run to raise money for "Kids in care". Good atmosphere and several people thanked me for joining in. We raised twice as much as we expected – we did something that mattered.	I made a difference to the charity. I matter to them. 6/8 I can take thanks and feel ok about it. 8/8
Sun evening	Exhausted again. Cancelled a date with Joe because I thought I needed to rest – but compromised by saying that I'd happily meet him in the week. He was ok about it.	It is important to look after myself and I can do this without upsetting others. 6/8 I should do this because I matter. 4/8

What I have learnt about myself over the week:
It's uncomfortable for me to accept compliments and to give myself credit (or to indulge myself) but the more I do this the easier it gets and the more I am inclined to believe that I do matter to others and that I can make a difference.
Now that I look out for thanks and compliments (and I don't dismiss them!) I realise just how much gratitude and praise that I used to ignore – paying attention to them boosts my self-esteem.

I believe:
"I matter" 4/8

Consider the following examples.

Rhiannon and her therapist had prepared for the BE, understood Rhiannon's fears, and come up with good reasons – and a good plan – for testing them. Now at the doorway of the supermarket, Rhiannon began to express a fear that she would have a panic attack. The therapist simply asked if Rhiannon could carry on, she did not explore the NAT. They had been over this very thoroughly and further exploration was unlikely to reveal any new understanding or solution and there was the risk that more discussion at this point would elevate her fear. The therapist also knew that Rhiannon was avoidant when stressed and did not want to collude with her in avoiding the BE – however, she did check with Rhiannon that it was okay to continue with the experiment.

Gerard's catastrophic thoughts and images just seemed to expand as his therapist probed more. Asking him questions like 'What could happen? What could go wrong?' and 'What would that mean to you?' seemed to take them deeper into catastrophisation. So, he and his therapist agreed that it was more productive to look at the process of worry and coping with worry rather than try to clarify the content of his fear and search for specific solutions.

Paula found that unpacking her thoughts and feelings with her therapist gave her a sense of order and safety, so she welcomed their verbal explorations. Knowing this, the therapist encouraged Paula to look at the pros and cons of being more 'Socratic-lite' at times.

SUMMARY

- Socratic methods *guide discovery* rather than *change minds*. In using Socratic methods in CBT we aim to ask, not to tell.
- Strategies can be predominantly verbal or behavioural (see Chapter 8).
- A Socratic intervention most often goes beyond a simple enquiry; many verbal Socratic strategies require well-structured dialogues.
- Logs and other self-monitoring activities add to our repertoire of Socratic techniques.
- A good Socratic intervention should be: hypothesis driven; answerable/doable; enlightening.
- Good Socratic practice is also knowing when *not* to use Socratic methods.

REFLECTION & ACTION

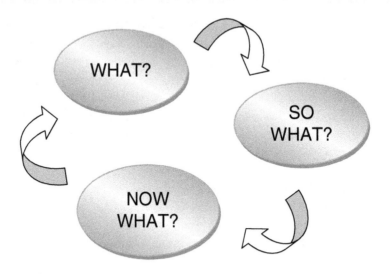

WHAT are you taking away from this chapter? What teaching points resonate with you?

....
....
....
....
....
....
....
....
....
....

SO WHAT? What significance do these points have – how do they relate to your previous learning or views? Do they challenge your former opinions? Have you gleaned new ideas for helping patients or indeed looking after your own needs?

....

....

....

....

....

....

....

....

....

....

NOW WHAT? How do you now plan to make the most of your Socratic skills? What are you now going to do differently? Make a commitment with yourself to follow through on at least one of your new ideas.

....

....

....

....

....

....

....

....

....

8

SOCRATIC METHODS: BEHAVIOURAL INTERVENTIONS

In 2019, at the World Congress of Behavioural and Cognitive Therapies, Dr Christine Padesky updated her 1993 keynote on Socratic method. She coined the phrase 'Action-packed CBT' to remind us that Socratic *method* should embrace much more than verbal techniques. We also use active strategies to yield new possibilities and perspectives, in particular behavioural experiments, surveys and logs, graded practice, role play and modelling. In this chapter, we look at each of these.

Of course, in CBT, behavioural tests have a *cognitive* rationale and *cognitive* review so this chapter makes an artificial distinction between the cognitive and the behavioural tasks. We routinely supplement experiential activities with verbal (Socratic) debriefing, especially if a person has difficulty in developing a new view. Following a behavioural experiment, we typically ask 'And what have you learnt?' and 'What will you do differently as a consequence?' In this way, we can be sure that there has been new learning and that this will manifest in new behaviour.

BEHAVIOURAL EXPERIMENTS

Behavioural experiments (BEs) in CBT are clearly and comprehensively explored in Bennett-Levy et al.'s (2004) book, but in summary they fall into different categories of planned, experiential, data-collecting activities:

- Observing something from scratch to collect data and kick start the process of developing hypotheses to test, perhaps through self-monitoring or carrying out surveys.

- Observing the behaviours of others to test hypotheses, perhaps by setting up surveys or simply planned people watching.
- Testing hypotheses by setting up personalised experiments such as bespoke graded exposure (and self-rating) to fearful situations or changing habitual behaviours to test the impact on others.

BEs are designed to generate evidence that can be used to refine and test a hypothesis. This can sound rather challenging until you consider that our hypotheses are simply the predictions or hunches that we routinely check out in CBT (see Table 8.1).

Sometimes we check our hunches by using Socratic enquiry, for example if I thought that a patient was depressed, I might start by asking questions and then perhaps augment this by administering a depression questionnaire. At this point the patient's answers could support or refute my hypothesis. I might then decide that I need yet more information and so engage in further Socratic exploration and negotiation of a BE to self-monitor.

The patient and I might initially explore 'I will fail in my presentation: I'll freeze' using verbal Socratic strategies, and we may indeed begin to shift the intensity of this belief but that shift might only be consolidated when they actively test out the prediction via a BE of giving a presentation and monitoring what happens.

Using BEs is different from applying Behaviour Therapy (BT), although BEs are derived from BT. If you are interested in this evolution, read Rachman's (2015) engaging and scholarly account of the shift and the distinctions between the approaches. The key difference is that BT is based on *exposure* leading to *habituation*, the natural diminishing of the fear response. Thus the premise is that if you stick it out the fear will pass and you will have a new learning experience, namely the feared event coupled with the sense of calm. I recall some successful experiences of this during my training as a clinical psychologist, particularly with the less 'psychologically-minded'.

On my very first training placement I worked with an elderly patient who held the belief that 'I'll panic in the shopping centre and fall or scream – it will be awful.' Together we devised a plan whereby I would take her to the centre and leave her for 15 minutes, during which

Table 8.1 Common predictions that can be tested

Common therapist predictions	Common patient predictions
This person is depressed	No-one will talk with me
There are problems at home	I will fail in my presentation: I'll freeze
This person doesn't understand flashbacks	I can't stand not knowing – I will go mad
This person will benefit from practising being assertive	There is nothing I can do to feel better
	I can't cope with being in the shopping centre
This person is at risk of self-harm	I can't be with people

time she would note her anxiety levels. I watched this frail, tiny woman from afar as she sat in a very busy public area – completely alone. What had I done?! After a quarter of an hour I approached her. I was a nervous wreck and she was fine. Within five minutes her anxiety had dropped, and she had spent most of the time feeling tranquil. At follow-up she was still using the mall and feeling okay about it: she had learnt a new response.

I have also worked with patients with a similar overarching prediction using BEs within CBT rather than exposure. Typically, we would devise a cognitive understanding of the fear, tease out negative predictions and then plan ways to test them. Below we can follow Vera through a BE-focused intervention.

Before we do so, an obvious question to consider is why choose BEs over exposure? Exposure seems less time-intensive and it can work. However, there is good indication that BEs are more effective, particularly in the long term, so it is worth the investment (for reviews see McMillan & Lee, 2010; Rachman, 2015).

A cognitive understanding of the problem

We identified Vera's fear-inducing beliefs and rated each of these (see below). We opted for a rating scale of 1–10 but this is something to be negotiated with each patient. Aim for precision in capturing cognitions as vague statements are hard to test. Vera began by saying 'I can't do shops.' Socratic dialogue helped to clarify what she meant with questions such as:

- 'What is that like for you, not being able to do shops?', 'What does that phrase mean?'
- 'If you had those feelings of not coping, what could happen?'
- 'And then what?'
- 'Is there anything else?'

Together we identified four relevant predictions (see Table 8.2).

Table 8.2 Vera's predictions

Prediction	Belief rating 0–10	How I cope
1. I can't stand the feelings of panic and fear in my local shop	9	Avoid the shop/take beta-blocker before going out
2. I will be overcome with fear and collapse	8	Avoid the shop and other scary places
3. People will think I'm weak and foolish	7	Avoid situations where I could collapse
4. No-one will help me	8	Avoid situations where I could collapse

The next Socratic intervention was simply asking 'Vera, when you look at this, what do you make of it?'. She replied that she realised she used avoidance to cope with fear and it was no wonder she never overcame her fear. Thus, we had a mini-formulation that gave us a rationale for intervening.

The next step in a BE is considering how to test the prediction (the hypothesis). As Vera's problem comprised several predictions there were several ways to take this forward, and you can see the different options below. However, all experiments:

- were devised collaboratively (with a shared rationale at their core);
- had evolved from the session;
- were set up as 'no-lose' – this is hypothesis testing, so whatever happens there will be 'data' to work with.

In session BE

Prediction 1:

With Vera's permission, this lent itself to a spontaneous BE. Vera could identify links between her fear of panic, over-breathing and increased panic symptoms: a vicious cycle. In session, we carried out preparatory work of learning controlled breathing (see Chapter 9) and she rapidly concluded that she could take charge of the symptoms of hyperventilation. This in itself resulted in a new belief ('I can manage unpleasant feelings') but she wanted to take it further so that she could be really confident about going out. Vera agreed to over-breathe in the session to trigger panic symptoms. The test was to stay with the feelings for one minute – and if this was too difficult, she could choose to ease her situation with controlled breathing. She brought on the panicky feelings and tried to stay with them for a minute, but she found that they kept diminishing unless she actively hyperventilated. This provided the experience needed for me to ask her 'What have you learned from this?' (see Table 8.3).

Armed with this experience, she felt sufficiently confident to take on Prediction 2.

Table 8.3 Prediction 1

Original prediction and belief rating	Test	New belief and rating
1. I can't stand the feelings of panic and fear 9/10	Evoke panicky feelings in session and stay with them for 1 minute	I can tolerate these feelings 8/10 I'm not afraid of these feelings 7/10 These feelings ease of their own accord 9/10 .... at least when I'm with my therapist in a clinic setting

In vivo BE

Prediction 2:

This real-life test carefully considered the how/what/where/when details so that Vera knew exactly what she needed to aim for. Vera deliberated on what might need to be in place to make the practice possible – she thought that walking to the shop alone would frighten her and leave her vulnerable to panic, so she would ask Bill to go with her. She also feared the busy lunch break and decided to shop before noon, and on a weekday as this would be quieter than Saturday. We planned carefully so that the task would challenge Vera without overwhelming her – it is generally best to avoid taking risks. She carried out the experiment and as agreed repeated it each day to consolidate her learning. At the end of the week we reviewed her experience (see Table 8.4).

The final column looks like a success story ('I will not collapse 8/10'), yet Vera's fear ratings remained high. This is not unusual with anxiety disorders because facing fears often brings on anxiety and so it is important to look at the behavioural changes and spot progress there. Vera was facing her fears and it was showing in her anxiety ratings.

Socratic enquiry also revealed that even though Vera now believed it was unlikely she would collapse, she said that *if* she did it would be unbearable because of predictions 4 and 5. This was maintaining high anxiety levels and we needed to address it.

Table 8.4 Prediction 2

Original prediction and belief rating	Specifics of the BE	Outcome	New belief and rating (end of week)
1. I will be overcome with fear and collapse 8/10	Go into local shop alone, at 11am on a weekday: Mon-Fri. Buy a pint of milk at self-service counter and leave. Rate fear 0-10. Walk there with Bill.	Day 1 & 2: Went ok – fear 7/10 Day 3: Bought five items. Went ok – fear 6/10 Day 4 & 5: Walked there alone. Went ok – fear 7/10	I can go to the local shop and feel reasonably calm 6/10 I will not collapse 8/10

Survey-based BE

Prediction 3:

I asked Vera what information she needed from others to test the validity of her prediction. She devised the following question: *'If you saw a woman in her 20s collapse in a small supermarket, what would you think of her?'* We then considered the ideal test population. She said that she wouldn't trust my colleagues to tell the truth because we were paid to be considerate, but she would trust her friends. She texted 12 friends (see Table 8.5).

Table 8.5 Prediction 3

Original prediction and belief rating	Test	Outcome	New belief and rating
1. People will think I'm weak and foolish 7/10	Text twelve friends with my question	12/12 would be concerned 6/12 would think that she might be ill 0/12 would think that she was weak or foolish	People wouldn't think me weak or foolish if I collapsed 8/10 People would be concerned 8/10

Vera said that she would now rate her fear of shopping as 5–6/10, which was an improvement but still quite high. Socratic review revealed that this was because she still believed that *if* she collapsed no-one would help her, and she had an upsetting image of lying on the floor with people stepping over her, not caring about her. So, this was the next prediction to be tackled.

Observational/modelling BE

Prediction 4:

Vera thought this could be tested if she actually collapsed and discovered how the public reacted, but she was emphatic that she would not take that risk. During pregnancy I had fainted so often that I was now fearless about dropping to the floor (possibly a triumph of exposure and habituation), so I offered to role play fainting in her local shop. Vera could then observe what happened. As before, we set up the task at a specific time in a particular (medium-sized) shop and Vera chose where I should collapse while she watched (see Table 8.6).

Table 8.6 Prediction 4

Original prediction and belief rating	Test	Outcome	New belief and rating
1. No-one will help me [Helen] 8/10	Helen will 'faint' near the checkout where there are always people.	Some people looked and walked on, but no-one ignored Helen and four or five came to her aid. They all expressed kind concern, offered her water and asked her if she wanted them to call an ambulance. No-one made too much of a fuss – I didn't feel embarrassed for her.	If I collapse someone will help me and will probably be discreet and kind 8/10

Vera now rated her fear of shopping as 4/10 and we were able to build on the cognitive shifts by setting up more challenging tasks. This was appropriate because it fitted with her overarching goal of being able to shop freely in the city, which specifically meant using the largest department store there at weekends. We approached this through graded steps (see next section).

Vera's BE experience was quite intensive, but it is worth noting that patients often benefit much more quickly. Often a single BE is trialed and patients, such as Phoebe and Johan (below), return to sessions able to summarise what they have learnt for themselves.

Phoebe took part in an active experiment on public transport: 'It was really hard to take that first step onto the coach but when I stepped off at the other end I just knew I could do this again; I knew that I'd be fine.'

Johan carried out a survey: 'By the time I'd asked the fifth person about their sleep pattern, I realised that I was well within the normal population. I relaxed.'

Graded tasks

A good general principle when helping patients tackle challenging activities is grade the task. Rather than attempting to achieve something in one go, build on manageable successes step by step. We reviewed this in Chapter 3 when we looked at goal setting, but it lends itself to a much wider range of activities that might otherwise overstretch our patients, for example:

- eating three balanced meals per day;
- completing a tax return;
- showering and teeth cleaning every day;
- getting through the day without checking their daughter's whereabouts;
- reading a textbook.

We use Socratic enquiry to define these challenges, break them down into manageable steps and review progress. Take the example of reading a textbook.

Jacob, a student, struggled with depressed mood and this affected his ability to concentrate and retain information. It transpired in therapy that he needed to be familiar with at least one of his core textbooks by the end of term. His (catastrophic) automatic thought was: 'I can't read a textbook in this state of mind. I'll never manage it. I'll disappoint my tutors and I'll get thrown off the course.'

His therapist asked information-gathering questions such as 'How long do you have until the end of term?', 'What has happened to other students who have not been able to complete this sort of assignment?', 'How long is the text?'. She then offered a summary to Jacob: 'It sounds as though one of the texts is shorter than the others, just 250 pages, and you could choose that one. We have nearly nine weeks to get through the book and when other students have not been able to complete similar assignments under similar conditions, the year tutor has always given them extra time and you think that you would get an extension. Have I understood this correctly? Hearing this – how does this sound to you?':

Jacob: It doesn't sound quite so hopeless.

Therapist: Given what's helped you in the past, do you have thoughts about tackling the assignment over the next eight weeks or so?

J: I could try to read small chunks of text, a bit at a time. But I'll just forget what I've read so that's no use.

Th: Is there anything you could do to help you remember the chunks of text that you have read?

J: Well the obvious thing is to make notes, I suppose.

Th: How does that strike you – reading a manageable amount of text and making notes as a memory jogger?

J: Sounds okay I suppose.

Th: Now – what do you think a manageable amount would be given what you know of your concentration and tiredness and what's the best time for you to do this reading? …

Together the therapist and Jacob detailed a series of steps that would be regarded as flexible:

- Plan: Read late morning/early afternoon when mood is a bit better and the fatigue hasn't set in. Rest and make notes at 15-minute intervals. Work for one hour at a time. Take weekends off.
  - Step 1: Aim to do one hour once or twice a week (and then do something active, if possible). Read notes before bed as a memory aid.
  - Step 2: Increase to 2–3 times per week.

  o Step 3: Increase to 3–4 times per week.

  o Step 4: Read for an hour each weekday.

Jacob gave himself a 'Hopeful' rating of 4/8.

  After the first week they reviewed progress – the therapist asked him (i) how things had gone, (ii) what he had learnt, (iii) how he might take things forward:

Jacob said that things had not gone well in that he found the textbook very dense and not easy to read – but he had then looked at one of the longer ones (320 pages) and found it more engaging so he had swapped books. From this he had learnt that he could be (and indeed should be) flexible. He had managed to spend an hour reading on three occasions and had made and reviewed his notes. From this he learnt that he was more capable than he had expected. So, his next step would be to increase to 4–5 reading sessions per week. He now saw that his 'all or nothing' view of managing assignments wasn't really working for him and that it was okay to take things a step at a time. His 'Hopeful' rating was 5/8.

  Jacob's experience is typical in that the plan is a work in progress and if each step stretches him without being overambitious it will do its job. When it was clear that the behavioural activity was overstretching him we devised ways to scale back the plan:

Therapist: So, reading for one hour each day wasn't possible this week – even though you had managed it in the previous week. That's interesting. What do you make of it?

Jacob: It was a tough week workwise and maybe it was too much to expect that I could read the textbook every day.

Th: Sounds reasonable – anything else?

J: Well I think that I really pushed myself last week because I wanted to get to Step 4, but I don't think I can keep up that sort of effort.

Th: That also makes good sense – no-one can stretch themself all the time. With hindsight – what have you learnt from your observations?

J: That I need to be realistic about what I can do. I need to resist the urge to achieve and I need to take stock and be flexible if necessary.

Th: What does 'being realistic' mean in practical terms?

J: It means dropping the high standards that put me at risk. I keep reminding myself: dare to be average.

Imagery can play a part in grading tasks as some demanding situations can be rehearsed in imagination before the in-vivo practice begins.

Courtney was so fearful of getting on the train that his graded practice began with him first imagining this. He and his therapist worked on a detailed script of the activity and she read it out as Courtney closed his eyes and tried to 'see' this as vividly as possible. Only when he had mastered this, did they move on to using a train in real life.

A final note about graded tasks – wherever possible, each step is best rehearsed until your patient feels comfortable. At that point the next step can be tackled. In this way we build on achievement and minimise risk-taking.

Theory A/Theory B

A particularly adaptable hypothesis-testing technique is the 'Theory A versus Theory B' strategy. This collaborative intervention, developed by Salkovskis and Bass (1997), offers the opportunity for collecting data to test two opposing theories. Although it was originally described to treat hypochondriasis it is extremely adaptable, and it is a beautifully Socratic technique as the patient generates the evidence, draws conclusions, and either reframes the problem or recognises the need to take this forward into problem-solving.

Essentially, Theory A is 'There is something bad' and Theory B is 'I am worrying too much about something bad':

- 'I'm seriously ill vs I'm OK, but I worry about having physical health problems and this makes me feel ill.'
- 'I'm boring vs I do have things to say but I panic in social situations and I clam up.'

We need to adopt a curious experimental approach to considering the two theories (see Table 8.7). Rather than proposing that a person is incorrect in holding a particular belief,

Table 8.7 Theory A/B

Event	Evidence for Theory A: I have bowel cancer.	Evidence for Theory B: My stomach pains and digestive problems are because I worry.
Sun: Wake up and need the loo urgently.	Irregular bowel habits are a sign of bowel cancer. This is common for me.	I was worrying about my health in the early hours of the morning. I felt quite normal for the rest of the day.
Mon: Stomach cramps in the afternoon.	Colonic pain is a sign of bowel cancer and this isn't the only time I've had pain.	The morning had been increasingly stressful, and my pain came on after a tense meeting. It disappeared when I got home.
Wed: Feeling nauseous all day.	Nausea is a sign of bowel cancer.	I was nervous about a presentation that I had to give at 4pm. I felt ok once it was over.

Conclusion & what I need to do: When my stress levels rise, I have more digestive problems: I am beginning to believe that I don't have cancer (6/10) but I have some doubt. There are lots of times when I'm not stressed or worried and I feel ok. I need to remind myself of this when I get stomach problems and I could also try to manage my stress during the day by taking time out to relax. I will continue to monitor this.

we ask them to consider that *perhaps* they are right but *perhaps* there is another possibility. These alternatives are then explored in therapy: Theory A reflects the client's predicted belief (e.g. 'I am seriously ill'), while Theory B states an alternative explanation (e.g. 'These symptoms are down to anxiety').

We can then test the theories both retrospectively (by reviewing past beliefs, behaviours and outcomes) and prospectively (by setting up behavioural tests). This both brings the benign theory into the client's awareness and potentially collects data to support it. We remain open to either theory being dominant.

We encourage patients to draw their own conclusions and consider how to take things forward – in some cases Theory A will be borne out and we will need to move forward to problem-solving. I recall this happening once (see Table 8.8) and therapy was adapted accordingly.

BEHAVIOURAL LOGS

An invaluable tool for data-collecting, and hypothesis-testing, is the activity schedule (often called the Weekly Activity Schedule: WAS). This is a simple grid first developed for monitoring

Table 8.8 Theory A/B

Event	Evidence for Theory A: My spouse is having an affair.	Evidence for Theory B: I am worried that Mike is having an affair and so I behave aggressively, and this is why our relationship is strained.
Wed: M phoned – he's staying at the hotel again tonight. Says it's work.	Phoned Liz and Trudy – their husbands are on their way back home.	I am nervous so I do think the worst and I feel aggressive towards Mike.
Conclusion & what I need to do: I'm not sure what's happening. I need to stay calm and call Karl the project manager. He will know what's going on at work.		
Wed: Karl said that they'd finished up the project today and everyone could go home.	Mike has lied to me.	I can't see it any other way right now.
Conclusion & what I need to do: I think I have a real problem in my marriage, it's not just me being paranoid after last time. I just want to drink and punch cushions but that doesn't do me any good. Instead I need to get myself support and start to think this through. I'm calling Jenna – she's a good friend who will talk straight and help me, and if she's not free I'll swallow my pride and ring mum – she does love me and she'll be on my side.		

and manipulating activity in depression (Beck et al., 1979) – but as we will see, it is so much more versatile.

Originally, patients were encouraged to complete a grid that captured an hourly snapshot of activity (see Tables 8.9 and 8.10). Using a 0–5 scale, they were asked to rate activity for:

- *pleasure*: This reflects positive feelings associated with an activity: how enjoyable something is. This is independent of …
- *mastery*: Beck et al. (1979) describe this as a sense of accomplishment. Such a notion can be difficult for some and so instead we often ask patients to note how difficult they found an activity. The higher the rating the more credit they can give themselves for carrying it out.

It has been suggested that the purposefulness of an activity is relevant in easing depression (Lejuez, Hopko, Acierno, Daughters & Pagoto, 2001, 2011), so it is worth considering adding another rating of purposefulness or meaningfulness that captures how worthwhile the activity seemed.

In the example below, walking might be rated as moderately pleasurable but very difficult, while watching TV was not difficult at all but gave very little pleasure. In reviewing a log, therapist and patient can explore the impact of an activity: 'How did you feel at the time? And what did you want to do? What happened then?'. This all helps to deepen an understanding

Table 8.9   Behavioural log: WAS

	Monday	Tuesday	Wednesday	Thursday	Friday	Saturday	Sunday
6.00–7.00							
7.00–9.00							
9.00–10.00							
10.00–11.00							
11.00–12.00							
12.00–1.00							
1.00–2.00							
2.00–3.00							
3.00–4.00							
4.00–5.00							
5.00–6.00							
6.00–7.00							
7.00–8.00							
8.00–9.00							
9.00–11.00							

of the patient's experiences and informs the formulation. Once patterns and links to pleasure and mastery have been identified, patients are encouraged to use these data to plan ahead to maximise pleasure in their lives.

There is an advantage to keeping the activity scheduling (AS) as simple as possible – a minimal entry of activity and a simple rating. However, if necessary, the basic template can be adapted for monitoring a wide range of thoughts, feelings or behaviours and it can be used for planning ahead to combat a wide range of difficulties. Nonetheless, we should be careful not to overload patients in our enthusiasm to better help them overcome their problems!

Table 8.10   Excerpt of WAS

12.00–1.00	Lunch alone P:2/M:0	Walking P3/M:5	Lunch alone P:3/M:0
1.00–2.00	TV P2/M:0	TV P2/M:0	Had to help in the shop P:2/M:5
2.00–3.00	Called Frankie P3/M:4	TV P1/M:0	Had to help in the shop P:3/M:4

A note about Behavioural Activation (BA) is probably relevant here: BA is well established as an effective treatment for some depressions. Like activity scheduling, it relies on structuring and scheduling. It differs from AS in that it is underpinned by functional analysis rather than collaborative conceptualisation and it does not focus on pleasant event scheduling. In 2013 Christopher Martel, a founder of BA, published an excellent paper that gives a comprehensive overview of BA and its practice, and it is well worth the read.

Activity scheduling in action
Monitoring

Vinnie was not very confident that CBT could help him. He couldn't say when and where he felt worse or better: 'I'm never free of a sense of threat and doom. It's why I drink and it's why I feel hopeless.' It was important to understand more about his experiences, so he and his therapist came up with the idea of keeping a record of his daily activities. This data-collecting exercise might allow them to see if his thoughts and feelings did fluctuate, to identify links between thoughts, feeling and behaviours. Vinnie had never kept a log like this (and he was sceptical of this being helpful) so they kept it as simple as possible and omitted ratings for the time being.

Below is an excerpt (see Table 8.11).

Vinnie's therapist reviewed the entire week's activities and comments. She asked Socratic questions such as 'You had thought that you were never free of the bad feelings: now you see your grid, how does it look to you?'. Vinnie was able to conclude *for himself* that his feelings and thoughts did fluctuate and that there might be patterns to this. For example, the more time he spent in bed and the more alcohol he drank at night the worse he felt. They developed the basis for building hypotheses that could be refined and/or tested.

At this point there are many options for taking things forward:

- The therapist could use some of the entries to help Vinnie see the links between thoughts, feelings and behaviours. These early stages of therapy psychoeducation and refining the formulation are key. They could build on the WAS by shifting to keeping a Thought Diary (see Chapter 7).
- They could focus on a specific prediction and test it, e.g. that Vinnie can only manage social situations with 'Dutch courage'. This would help him develop the essential skill of

Table 8.11 Activity Record

	Monday What happened: how did I feel/think/act?	Saturday What happened: how did I feel/think/act?
	Activity Record	
7.00–8.00	Get up, shower, breakfast: no time to think. Feel OK.	Lying in bed.
8.00–9.00	Drive to work, listening to radio (news): no time to think. Feel OK.	Bit hungover. Angry with myself for drinking so much last night.
9.00–10.00	Teaching new staff to use new IT equipment. Self-conscious. Worried I'm boring/stupid.	Tired but can't get back to sleep. Feel dreadful – worried and have bad feeling in pit of stomach.
10.00–11.00	Monthly departmental meeting – ok at first but as it went on, I got lost in my thoughts and was quiet. Felt stupid and thought that it's always going to be like this for me – never good enough. I hate myself.	Get up, shower, breakfast. Feel a bit better but still can't shake off the gloom and doom. Worried about meeting J for picnic lunch – she'll just be bored by me.
11.00–12.00		Walked into town to get pub lunch by myself – needed the air. This helped a bit. Had a drink.
12.00–1.00	In town bought some wine to take to lunch. Still worried. Had a vodka for Dutch courage: I can't manage without it.	Lunch went better than I expected. J brought the puppy and we walked him through the park. We didn't drink the wine because J was driving, and I still managed to laugh a bit and J did too. We said we'd do this again soon.
1.00–2.00	Solitary paperwork. Feeling embarrassed for needing to drink in the middle of the day. Feel ashamed that I'm so weak and useless	

behavioural experimentation and perhaps also give him the motivation to try to break free of the 'drinking trap' (see the earlier section on BEs).

- They could continue to build on the skills that Vinnie could develop through using the grid (decentring, clarifying thoughts, feelings and behaviours, identifying patterns). By now introducing mood or cognition ratings could help him refine his evaluation. This would enable him to become more precise, to combat dichotomous responses, and it would also help him better appreciate change and progress.

- They could also introduce new ratings – pleasure, purposefulness and difficulty – so that Vinnie could begin to see what cheered him, what gave him a sense of meaningful achievement, and he could give himself credit for doing something difficult.

The formulation is an invaluable aid in deciding how to progress. If Vinnie's therapist was aware that they still struggled with their collaborative development of maintaining cycles, she might opt for the first option as it would generate more details of patterns and linkages. If the 'drinking trap' was a prominent issue, which related to Vinnie's therapy goals, then option 2 might be the way to go.

Together they decided to gather more detailed information by building on the grid. Vinnie now had the hang of noting his activities and felt that he could manage to add in ratings. Its next format included precise ratings that were negotiated with Vinnie so that his language was used (Enjoyable, Purposeful, Difficult). He felt that he could discriminate using a 0–5 scale (more than this seemed overwhelming to him) so that scale was adopted. They also agreed that it would be helpful to add an 'Urge to drink' rating as Vinnie wanted to tackle his alcohol consumption. A sample of Vinnie's log is shown in Table 8.12.

Adding the ratings to the log really taxed Vinnie – he couldn't imagine having to do this every day. But he kept going because his therapist had explained that this was a temporary exercise that would give them a better understanding of his problems. Together they reviewed his recent log and again Vinnie's therapist asked questions such as 'When you look at this, do you see patterns?', 'Do you notice links?'. In this way she again helped Vinnie to draw his own conclusions about his behaviours, thoughts, feelings and urges. For example, he saw that it was effortful to meet up with a friend, but it always raised his mood, especially if he and the friend did something purposeful like help out at the local food bank. She also asked what he had learnt overall from carrying out the exercise, and he said that he had learnt that things do make sense if you look closely and that meant that he was less hard on himself: he felt less stupid when he struggled.

Planning

WAS monitoring provides a rich database for the next stage – planning. It becomes clear what activities improve affect and give a sense of purpose (and in Vinnie's case what makes him prone to drinking). Thus, the following week can be timetabled to be as therapeutic as possible.

Table 8.12 Activity Record with ratings

Activity Record

Monitor what happens each day and rate your reactions using the following scale:

Absent			Moderate		Strong
0	1	2	3	4	5

- How I felt (0–5)
- What went through my mind: how much I believed it (0–5)
- How ENJOYABLE I found the activity (E: 0–5)
- How meaningful/PURPOSEFUL it seemed (P: 0–5)
- How DIFFICULT it was for me at the time (D: 0–5)
- My URGE to drink (U: 0–5)

Time	Monday What happened: how did I feel/think/act?	Saturday What happened: how did I feel/think/act?
7.00–8.00	Get up, shower, breakfast: no time to think. Feel OK (3/5) E: 1 P:2 D:5 U: 0	Lying in bed: no hangover(!) E: 4 P:4 D:0 U: 0
8.00–9.00	Drive to work, listening to radio (music): no time to think. Feel OK (3/5) E: 3 P:2 D:3 U: 0	"Can't face the day – too much of a challenge": 4/5 Feeling glum: 4/5 "Good to have no hangover, though": 5/5 E: 1 P:1 D:1 U: 0
9.00–10.00	Administration; "This is dull, I'm slow and it makes me feel worse" 5/5 I feel so hopeless and miserable 4/5 E: 0 P:4 D:5 U: 4	Forced myself to get up and shower "Perhaps I can do something with the day" 3/5 Feeling less glum: 3/5 E: 1 P:2 D:4 U: 3
10.00–11.00	Meeting to discuss my ideas about developing a product. "This will go down like a lead balloon" 4/5 I feel pessimistic and miserable 4/5 – Positive response to my proposal! "I do have good ideas!" 4/5 and now I feel good 4/5 E:3 P:5 D:5 U: 0	Supermarket shop: "I am doing something with my day" 4/5 Feeling less glum: 3/5 "I want to buy a bottle of vodka – I need it" 4/5 … but I resist and feel good about it 4/5 E: 1 P:4 D:5 U:5

Vinnie's therapist guided him in planning and problem-solving and creating his new schedule by asking what might be enjoyable or purposeful. This helped to not only shape Vinnie's planned activities but also refined his ideas for his overarching therapy goals. He found the prospect of planning for a whole week rather daunting, so his therapist asked what might make it easier and he said not having to do this every day. Therefore, he and his therapist agreed that they'd run an experiment whereby he carefully scheduled one day but not the next and so on. Before Vinnie put his plans into action, his therapist helped him to *troubleshoot*.

Once you have evolved plans, always anticipate and prepare for obstacles to progress. Patients need to be prepared and flexible, so ask questions such as:

- 'I think this is a good plan but just to be on the safe side let's consider, what could go wrong?'
- 'How might you prepare yourself/deal with this if it happened?'
- 'How might a friend prepare themself/deal with this if it happened?'
- 'What would we learn from that?'
- 'So, can you now sum up your back-up plans?'

Vinnie and his therapist met a week later and reviewed his experiences. Each activity, each day and the week as a whole had provided valuable learning, e.g. he learnt that he could in fact exert some control over his life and his feelings, that his mood was better and more stable on the days that he planned, that he could tolerate more social contact than he had predicted. He also realised that he had been overzealous in some respects (such as planning to go jogging before work) and this led to a review of his planning that embraced a graded return to exercise. He was comfortable about accommodating obstacles because of the preparatory work he'd done with his therapist.

Vinnie had ensured that his experiences had provided learning opportunities by consistently reviewing the outcome and being flexible – a necessary life skill for our patients.

ENACTING

Role play and rehearsal

A very versatile and necessary experiential strategy in our CBT armoury is role play. At assessment, enactment of challenging situations can enhance a Socratic review.

Abe, a student, struggled to catch the cognitions that made him so fearful of speaking in class. So, his therapist asked him if they might role play this. They agreed on a semi-formal activity (he would present a summary of his research ideas) and they enacted this in-session. After just a minute his therapist paused and asked 'How are you feeling right now?'. 'Terrified!' was the answer. She then asked 'Can you tell me what's going through your mind?', and Abe was now easily able to access a string of NATs.

Role play can also form an invaluable part of treatment. A new way of behaving can be rehearsed and enacted in the safety of the therapy session and learning opportunities reviewed. Typically, the patient will undertake the following:

1. *Role play*: patient as self, therapist as 'other' – thus giving insights into the patient's struggle, as with Abe. However, there are other options – see Brit below.
2. *Discussion*: how the patient feels they need to be able to behave, which leads to planning a new behaviour.
3. *Role play*: therapist modelling the new way of behaving.
4. *Debriefing*: what the patient has learnt from role play and how this might inform their own behaviour in the next role play.
5. *Role play(s)*: patient as themself taking on the new way of being – this can be repeated and debriefed as often as necessary.
6. *Debrief(s)*: patient reviews what they have learnt from the role play and how this can inform their behaviour.
7. *Between-session assignment*: usually to enact the role play in real life – this needs a sound rationale, careful planning and troubleshooting.

Brit tearfully described how she couldn't bring herself to counter her son's cruel comments because she was overwhelmed by anger and hurt. The therapist took on the role of the patient whilst Brit played the teenage son who had been so harsh. After the role play, without prompting, Brit said that she'd begun to realise how frustrated and confused her son must be and this helped her to feel empathy rather than anger. She said that she needed to be assertive with her son in drawing a line about acceptable and unacceptable comments and she and her therapist came up with a statement:

'Finn, I do understand that the way we live frustrates you, but I want more harmony in the household. This will benefit us all now that dad has gone, and we are all struggling. I am happy to hear your worries and to listen to what you want to change but from now on I'm drawing a line when your comments hurt me. I'm just going to walk away. This doesn't mean that I don't love you – I will always love you – but I am not going to stay in the room to be hurt. I think that is best for all of us.'

First, her therapist spoke these words and Brit played Finn. In doing so, Brit realised that she was happy with what she would say to her son so the role play shifted to Brit making her assertive statement while the therapist passively played Finn. Following a debrief where they decided that it would be more realistic if 'Finn' were argumentative, they carried out another role play where the therapist interrupted and insulted Brit. This gave Brit an opportunity to practise saying: 'I'm walking away now but I'm happy to talk later.'

She and her therapist role played and debriefed until Brit felt confident (8/10) that she could respond to Finn in a calm and assertive way and at this point they planned a between-session assignment to do just that.

In this example the role play incorporated rehearsal but sometimes we can spontaneously attempt rehearsal and then reflect on the learning and action opportunities:

Ken said that he'd like to be able to decline invitations for social drinks after work and his therapist invited him to have a go using her as a stooge. For him simply practising the statement in the session gave him sufficient confidence to try it out in real life.

Modelling

While it can be argued that modelling itself is a didactic teaching method, it can be part of a Socratic process because of the post-modelling review.

Jody struggled to be assertive. She could not yet face the first task in her graded practice, which was to make eye contact with, and give a compliment to, the person who served her in the department store. So, her therapist modelled doing this in a local shop: he bought a small item, smiled at the sales assistant and said 'Thank you for being so very helpful.' He then asked Jody the Socratic question:

'What did you take from watching me?'. Jody was able to say that she had been surprised at how quick and easy the interaction had been and how comfortable the sales assistant was with the smile and the compliment. She said that she now felt that she could copy the behaviour of the therapist herself. They then devised a plan to do that.

Modelling can be a powerful technique and over the years I have had to grit my teeth and hold all manner of insects and poke all manner of substances, but it is worth it because it helps patients. I've lost count of the number of times a patient has taken a spider from me because they have seen me holding it, or who had dared to approach a dog because they have watched me pet it first. As with all behavioural interventions, activities need to be negotiated so that the timing is right. My holding a spider or petting a dog would not be helpful if witnessing this overwhelmed the patients and simply re-enforced 'I can't cope with this.'

SUMMARY

- Socratic methods extend to behavioural interventions. Socratic conversation is crucial in setting up behavioural tasks and debriefing them.
- Behavioural experiments can take several forms but they must be well-planned and carefully evaluated – otherwise you risk losing valuable learning opportunities.
- Behavioural logs not only give us useful data but also serve as a Socratic medium for patients to draw new conclusions and plan new actions.
- Tasks are often best graded so that the patient is stretched but not overstretched.
- Enacting new ways of being either through role play or rehearsal can help to build confidence as well as offering a safe way of learning more about obstacles to change.
- Modelling can be used to prepare patients for change by offering an opportunity to observe, learn and adapt their way of being.

REFLECTION & ACTION

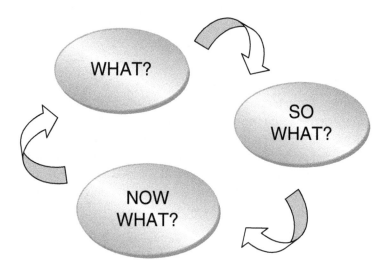

WHAT are you taking away from this chapter? What teaching points resonate with you?

....

....

....

....

....

....

....

....

....

....

SO WHAT? What significance do these points have – how do they relate to your previous learning or views? Do they challenge your former opinions? Have you gleaned new ideas for helping patients or indeed looking after your own needs?

....

....

....

....

....

....

....

....

....

....

NOW WHAT? How will you now use your Socratic skills to best advantage? What are you now going to do differently? Make a commitment with yourself to follow through on at least one of your new ideas.

....

....

....

....

....

....

....

....

....

9

YOUR BASIC CBT 'TOOLKIT'

Every CBT therapist will build a versatile 'toolkit' comprising generic and transdiagnostic strategies. These will comprise first principles of CBT and highly specific techniques.

I've used the term 'toolkit', but as Beck and colleagues remind us (Hofmann, Asmundson & Beck, 2013), CBT is much more than a collection of techniques and strategies, and CBT therapists are much more than technicians. We carefully select particular strategies in response to a psychological understanding of a person's problems (a formulation), and we do this in an empirical fashion (developing and testing hypotheses and collecting data for review).

We are the tourist who understands the culture and speaks the language, rather than the one who just gets by with a phrase book.

FUNDAMENTAL TOOLS

Many CBT techniques are truly transdiagnostic, fit for purpose for a number of disorders. Thus, you will have a set of skills that will stand you in good stead across a range of psychological problems. Most fundamentally, you will know how to *establish a working alliance* (Chapter 2) and that alone can be therapeutic for some patients. Just as important, you can assess problems and build a *collaborative conceptualisation* of a person's difficulties, creating a framework that embraces aetiology and maintaining cycles (Chapter 5). In doing this you are introducing *psychoeducation* and you will be able to judge if a patient's problem is appropriate for CBT and if indeed your patient is open to CBT at this time. Crucially, you can *identify vicious cycles* or 'traps' that will maintain difficulties and also direct you towards interventions. In addition you are spotting *virtuous cycles* of strengths, resources and coping skills.

Some of the 'traps' will be driven by cognitive factors – cognitive biases, intrusive images, automatic thoughts and core beliefs – and you are now in a position to identify these. Similarly, you can identify the behavioural drivers: avoidance, inactivity, reassurance-seeking and so on.

By now you know how to help patients monitor their difficulties and compile relevant information (e.g. using a thought record), so that the elements of the traps can be detailed. In doing so you make the generic vicious cycle bespoke, and also detailing the traps opens up a world of intervention possibilities because each 'staging point' in a vicious cycle points to possible strategies. For example:

Leone heard that there was a department party at the end of the month, and she felt scared. 'What if I go and no-one wants to talk? No-one will want to talk with me. What if I don't go and people think badly of me? Either way I'm a useless failure. Two weeks to go – I can't stand this waiting. I need a drink.'

Here the generic cycle has been personalised with Leone's particular experience and now a tailored intervention can be devised. But this must be informed by what we know of

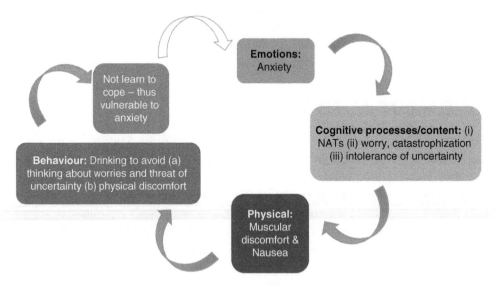

Figure 9.1 Leone's anxiety trap

best practice. For example, if we look at the *cognitive processes/content* element of the trap, there are many options for moving forward. We could focus on NATs, helping Leone identify the cognitive biases in the thoughts: 'No-one will want to talk with me/I'm a useless failure.' Or we could systematically review them using a thought record, or we could use metaphor, asking her to consider what her best friend would say to her, or we could devise a survey whereby she gathered information from friends to test her views. The choice will be determined by the stage of therapy, what research tells us and patient resources. We could also explore the metacognitions associated with worry, or we could teach distraction so that Leone could opt to put her worries to one side, we could help her develop her use of problem-solving skills to better resolve her worry – what we wouldn't do is focus on the content of the worry and we wouldn't encourage distraction if Leone used this as an SSB.

As you go through this chapter, look back at the trap and consider your options to help Leone manage the problem cognitions, physical symptoms or the unhelpful behaviours.

You also know how to guide patients in *decentering* when distressed and in *reviewing key cognitions*, and if necessary, testing these via *behavioural experiments*. You know how to progress to *problem-solving* when that is most appropriate. You have many talents.

Crucially, you can use Socratic enquiry to review what a patient concludes from their new experience and how they feel. In this way you check that the techniques are being used as coping strategies and not as safety-seeking behaviours, and that the outcome is targeting relevant affect and is not simply an intellectual exercise.

There is even more in the CBT toolkit. Below is a collection of particularly versatile techniques.

Physical techniques

This family of strategies includes controlled breathing and relaxation, but physical strategies do not just focus on calming, they also include applied tension and exercise for those times when getting active or raising blood pressure is necessary.

These physical techniques can be invaluable in breaking free of traps driven by:

- *excessive tension and over-breathing* – e.g. in anxiety disorders such as panic disorder and generalised anxiety disorder, or in anger management problems;
- *a lack of tension and lowered blood pressure* – e.g. in blood phobia;
- *inactivity* – e.g. in depression.

Controlled breathing and relaxation

This section presents an overview of each of these approaches, but you can also download a script for guiding patients through breathing and relaxation exercises by going to the OCTC webpage at www.octc.co.uk/wp-content/uploads/2016/07/Relaxation-scripts.pdf.

Breathing might seem like a strange skill to teach as we can all breathe, but controlled breathing is a technique that comes into play when a person over-breathes or *hyperventilates*. We tend to breathe more rapidly when we are stressed or exercising and this is not troublesome in the short term, in fact rapid breathing provides muscles with oxygen to prepare the body for action. However, continued rapid breathing can cause physical discomforts, such as tingling face and hands, muscle tremor or pain, lightheadedness, breathing difficulties. Understandably, this can be frightening and therefore heighten anxiety – a simple but powerful trap (see Figure 9.2).

Fortunately, it is relatively easy to learn how to counter over-breathing and break out of the trap. Patients simply need to respond to hyperventilation by respiring gently and evenly (preferably nasally), filling the lungs, before exhaling slowly. This avoids the 'shallow breathing' (breathing from the upper chest alone) or gulping that can actually worsen hyperventilation. In the early stages we would encourage patients to lie or sit whilst getting used to the sensations of controlled breathing. Once this rhythmic respiration is comfortable and familiar, they can try it in less relaxing settings such as when walking through town or sitting in a cinema etc. As with many coping strategies, the skill develops with practice, so the more repetitions the better.

Once controlled breathing can be used at will, it can be brought into play to break the cycle of tension and over-breathing.

Not only do we tend to hyperventilate when we are stressed or afraid, but also the muscles in our bodies tense. This is an automatic reaction, perfectly normal, and it prepares us for action. But in excess this too can cause uncomfortable sensations such as a headache, neck, shoulder or chest pain, breathing problems, trembling, a racing heart, churning stomach, tingling in the hands and face. As you might expect, any of these sensations can be worrying and could therefore increase muscular tension – another powerful trap (see Figure 9.3).

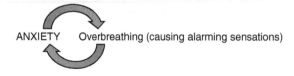

ANXIETY   Overbreathing (causing alarming sensations)

Figure 9.2

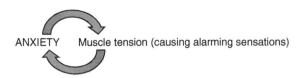

ANXIETY   Muscle tension (causing alarming sensations)

Figure 9.3

An effective way of managing bodily tension is through physical relaxation. Relaxing is more than sitting in front of the television or having a hobby (although these recreations are important too). *Really* relaxing requires the skill of reducing unnecessary physical tension whenever necessary and in a variety of situations.

This skill does not necessarily come easily and it needs to be practised. Like controlled breathing, it is often best learnt by progressing through a series of structured exercises. Usually we begin with some general guidelines advising patients to plan and evaluate their relaxation practice: deciding when and where will be quiet and comfortable. All exercises begin with a breathing check to ensure even and rhythmic respiration and they end with a gentle resuming of normal activities.

Then we introduce a series of routines designed to teach relaxation step by step. Typically, there are four stages, but this can be adapted to the person.

Stage 1: Systematic muscular relaxation

These exercises require a person to tighten and then relax muscle groups within the body in a systematic fashion. Usually, instructions are given to (gently) tense and then relax the feet, lower legs, upper legs, torso, arms, shoulders and neck, face.

The routine helps the very tense begin to distinguish between taut and relaxed muscles and to learn to recognise muscular tension and relax in response to this. Repeated practice is necessary but once relaxation is reliably achieved, Stage 2 can be introduced.

Stage 2: Short systematic relaxation

Stage 1 can be shortened by simply missing out the 'tense' stage. This modified exercise needs to be rehearsed, and when it is effective it can be adapted for use at other times and in other places (e.g. in a less quiet room) so that the skill is increasingly adapted to real life.

Stage 3: Simple relaxation routine

This is an even shorter exercise, suitable for those who can achieve a relaxed state with minimal guidance. It requires a person to sit in a comfortable position, allowing their body to become heavy and their breathing to become gentle and regular. On each in-breath, a sooth-ing word or mental picture is brought to mind, and on each out-breath, the sense of relaxation and heaviness is intensified.

Stage 4: Cued relaxation

Once stages 1 to 3 become effective the relaxation skills can be cued throughout the day and not just practised at designated relaxation times. In response to a prompt (e.g. a discreet alarm on a phone or a watch) a person simply:

> drops their shoulders;
> untenses muscles in the body;
> checks their breathing;
> relaxes;
> moves on.

Thus, relaxation becomes a portable skill to be used when needed.

It can be helpful to keep a record as it encourages reflective review and ensures that pro-gress does not go unnoted (see Table 9.1 for a typical relaxation record).

It is only natural to have the odd occasion when it is not possible to achieve a relaxed state, and the usual suspects are trying too hard, not being in a place conducive to relaxing, not being well rehearsed enough, catching the hyperventilation or tension too late for effective management. When a patient struggles simply help them to review what got in the way of easy relaxation and then shift to planning how to overcome obstacles in the future.

Although most patients benefit from beginning with the lengthy exercise and gradually reducing it, some people would prefer to start with the simple routine.

George had been abused as a child and now feared letting down his guard, so his therapist sug-gested starting with the simple relaxation exercise that allowed him to remain sitting with his eyes open. In this way George remained aware of what was happening in his environment and thus he felt in control. As he grew more confident that it was safe for him to relax, his therapist encouraged him to try the deeper relaxation exercises.

Table 9.1 Relaxation record

Relaxation record

Monitor your progress by rating your level of relaxation before and after carrying out a relaxation exercise. You can use the following scale:

Not relaxed Tense			Moderately relaxed			Very relaxed		
0	1	2	3	4	5	6	7	8

Date/Time	Type of exercise	Rating before	Rating after	Notes
Wed 10am	Systematic Muscular Relaxation	7	3	Quite helpful – better than last time (I think I might be getting the hang of it). Did notice the cold so I'll use a blanket next time I'm lying down to relax.
Sat 6pm	Systematic Muscular Relaxation	7	7	What bad timing: TV blaring in next room, me thinking about getting supper rather than let my worries go. I will plan better next time – I realise that I can't just squeeze this into a busy day.
Sun 11am	Short Systematic Relaxation	7	2	I'm getting better at this. I could really let my worries and tension drift away today as I sat in the easy chair. All the practice pays off.
Wed noon	Simple relaxation	6	4	Sitting at home. Quite easy to do this after all the practice with the longer exercises. It felt natural and it helped that I had lovely memories of walking along the beach on our last holiday.
Sat 11am	Simple relaxation	8	4	Tense in the house because of all the bickering. Went up to my bedroom for a few minutes and was able to get calm and then face the family again.
Fri 8 pm	Cued relaxation	6	4	Needed to relax before dinner in a public place – went to loo and spent a minute letting the tension leave my body while I got my breathing nice and smooth. It took the edge off my tension.

147

Applied tension and exercise

Sometimes problems occur because of low blood pressure. We see this, for example, in people who grow faint when they see, or anticipate seeing, blood or in those whose post-traumatic reaction is one of faint rather than fight or flight.

Janice had become quite reclusive because she disliked the woozy feeling she sometimes experienced when she went out. She feared that she might faint and hurt or embarrass herself so now she tended to stay at home. Her doctor explained that she had low blood pressure, like other members of her family, and that she could learn to tense her muscles, raise her blood pressure (BP) and manage the unpleasant sensations.

Phil had always felt faint on seeing blood and he'd become quite phobic about blood and even needles. His therapist explained that it is normal for BP to drop when we see blood and this could easily cause feelings of faintness. To counter this, she taught Phil to use applied tension, which quite quickly restored his confidence and the extreme fear disappeared.

Teaching applied tension is simply a matter of adapting the exercises above so that the focus is only on tensing muscles and developing the skill of doing this even when feeling woozy. Generally, this is combined with controlled breathing to minimise the likelihood of dizziness from hyperventilation (Gilchrist & Ditto, 2012).

Finally, physical exercise can play an important part in a patient's recovery. It has long been established that physical activity helps people break free from inactivity that fuels low mood or anxieties by reducing a sense of achievement and purposefulness. Physical activity also stimulates the brain to produce some of the 'feel-good' bio-chemicals (Kvam, Lykkedrang Kleppe, Nordhus & Hovland, 2016; Mikkelsen, Stojanovska, Polenakovic, Bosevski & Apostolopoulos, 2017).

Thus, the vicious cycle shown in Figure 9.4 is broken.

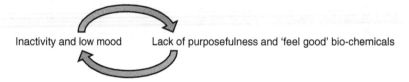

Inactivity and low mood   Lack of purposefulness and 'feel good' bio-chemicals

Figure 9.4

A very well-established technique for increasing physical activity is Behavioural Activation (BA), which uses highly-structured activity scheduling and review (see Chapter 8). A simpler intervention is simply taking steps to incorporate regular exercise and purposeful activity into daily life – and monitoring the impact of this, of course.

Kyle had grown less active as his mood dipped. Through behavioural monitoring and behavioural experiment, he realised that even small increases in his social activity raised his spirits, and doing even minor tasks around the house bolstered his sense of worth.

Simple cognitive techniques

As you have seen, in CBT we use cognitive review and testing (see Chapters 7 and 8), but we also use other, relatively simple cognitive techniques.

Decentring

A fundamental cognitive technique is *decentring*, the action of standing back and seeing a thought or image as just that – a mental event, not necessarily a truth. We can also decentre and consider a feeling as just a feeling.

For some this detachment and review is enough to get a new and less distressing perspective. For others, decentring coupled with recognising cognitive bias (see Chapter 1) does the trick.

A self-critical thought instantly brought down Harvey's mood and then he remembered to mentally stand back from the cognition and label it 'just a thought.' The thought instantly had less emotional impact even though it remained an unpleasant notion

Moira's anxiety rose: 'He thinks I'm an absolute fool.' Then she took a moment to decentre, feel calmer and then rethink. She concluded 'Hang on, I'm mind reading again and jumping to a conclusion. Actually, I've no idea what he's thinking.' She immediately felt some relief.

Addie usually concluded 'I feel scared so something must be wrong.' Decentring led him in a different direction. He learnt to drop his shoulders, breathe evenly, and say 'I feel scared but that's just a feeling. A feeling is not a fact.' By doing this he calmed himself and began to build a database, which supported the notion that feeling an emotion could be independent of, or even at odds with, reality.

Distraction

A more demanding yet still conceptually simple strategy is distraction. Based on the premise that we can only fully concentrate on one thing at once, distraction helps to reduce our distress by shifting our attention to something neutral or positive. This means it is possible to break free of the trap of negative cognitions (thoughts or images) fueling our negative mood, which in turn drives negative thinking (see Figure 9.5).

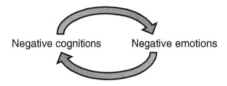

Figure 9.5

The key to successful distraction lies in:

- devising tasks that grab attention (use your patients' interests);
- keeping tasks specific – vague tasks tend not to be so effective;
- having several strategies for different settings because not all techniques will fit all settings (see Table 9.2 below);
- practice, practice, practice.

There are three basic distraction techniques.

1. Physical exercise

Keeping active when distressed so that it is difficult to dwell on upsetting thoughts. The simpler the activity the easier it can be to engage, so don't underestimate the impact of a short walk or clearing out a cupboard or even organising a handbag or briefcase. Your patients will need to experiment to find a few physical activities that will work for them in different situations – going jogging is not always possible!

Table 9.2 Distraction techniques

Anxiety provoking situation(s)	Suitable distraction technique
Sitting in the bus shelter	Read car number plates Listen to soothing music through ear buds Attend to my breathing and talk myself through a simple relaxation exercise
Waiting in the hospital	Review my photographs on my phone Play Solitaire on phone Read my novel Watch others come and go and try to guess their occupation
At home, worrying about my health	Go for a run Do some gardening (favourite hobby) Clear out the airing cupboard Watch gardening programmes on TV/DVD
In bed at night, frightened	Do a long relaxation exercise Remember my recent visit to a National Trust Garden in detail, remembering the smells and the sounds as I recall walking through the gardens

2. Refocusing

Paying great attention to things around, such as: counting the number of men or women with blonde or short hair; looking for certain objects in a shop window; studying the details of someone's outfit or a picture; reading the small print on tins in the supermarket; noticing the smells and sounds in the environment. The task doesn't need to be sophisticated but it does need to be absorbing, and the more detailed the task the more distracting it will be.

3. Mental exercise

This requires more creativity and mental effort. It might involve reciting some poetry or a piece of music, recalling a favourite holiday trip in detail, practising mental arithmetic, studying someone nearby and trying to guess what they do, dwelling on an imaginary scene and so on. The latter are more effective if they come alive with colour, sounds and texture, and if they suit the patient's preferences. There is no point in dwelling on a picture of a sun-soaked beach if we hate the sea and sunburn easily, or if our real love is skiing. A better mental picture would be of a snow-covered mountainside and a journey down a particularly satisfying slope.

Strategies need to be practised and refined and even so there will be times when they are not very effective. This might be for several reasons:

- More practice is needed.
- The technique didn't fit the situation.
- Initial stress levels were very high or the situation itself was stressing.
- Distraction is used as a safety-seeking behaviour (see Salkovskis, Clark, Hackmann, Wells and Gelder, 1999 for a description). Do always debrief to ensure that the patient appreciates success as an indication of them being able to take command of a situation so that their confidence grows.

Simple imagery work

Problem images can be identified in virtually all the disorders that we work with and much has been written on imagery work since the inception of CBT. An excellent reference for imagery work is *Imagery in cognitive therapy* written by Hackmann, Bennett-Levy and Holmes (2011). This is a comprehensive handbook that goes beyond basic CBT, but the authors remind us that very simple visual techniques can still make a difference. Using imagery does not need to be challenging for therapist or patient.

Rehearsing in imagination has been shown to increase the perceived plausibility of an event happening (Szpunar and Schacter, 2013), which means that it can enhance confidence, and it has been shown that mental images can evoke similar physiological and emotional responses to the real thing (Pearson, Clifford & Tong, 2008). Thus, we can usefully integrate imagery into therapy in order to:

- *build confidence*, step by step, in those not yet ready to face challenges in real life, e.g. a patient with a fear of snakes holding increasingly challenging mental images of snakes as a prelude to visiting the local zoo and handling one in vivo;
- *substitute* when it is not possible to practise in real life, e.g. someone with a fear of flying repeatedly imagining themselves travelling by plane – for financial and practical reasons it would not have been possible to repeat this experience in real life;
- *prepare* to take on a challenge, e.g. a patient imagining themselves walking into a public area feeling calm – reviewing this image helped them to feel calmer and more confident when they took on a social task for real.

We have already seen how mental images can enhance distraction; Beck et al. refer to using 'visual imagery as a diversion from dysphoria' back in 1979 (p. 172) and Beck and colleagues describe many simple imagery techniques for managing anxiety disorders (1985). More recently there has been a focus on image management in post-traumatic conditions (e.g. Ehlers and Clark, 2000) and you can download an OCTC document that summarises understanding traumatic intrusions from www.octc.co.uk/wp-content/uploads/2016/10/Understanding-traumatic-intrusions-OCTC-practical-guide.pdf.

Some problem visualisations will diminish simply as a result of understanding and formulating them (see Chapter 5) while others will persist. Persistent images can be managed in several ways.

Distraction

Alana struggled with the urge to drink – the visual image of a glass of wine and the bodily sensation of its cool taste and relaxing effect played on her mind as she walked through the shops. She was so tempted. Then she shifted her attention to the lyrics of a song that she knew well, and recalling the song not only displaced the image but also cheered her and reduced her stress

Holding the image and manipulating it to change its emotional impact

Brandon's memory of being threatened at work kept returning. It was vivid and disturbing, but he learnt to accept that it might come back and when it did, he imagined the customer who threatened him shrinking into a child and the knife that he held turning into a harmless soft toy. Then the child was led away by a kindly police officer. Brandon noted that his feelings changed, the intense fear subsided, and he felt safe. Soon the images reduced in frequency and intensity.

Charlotte was low and hopeless about ever losing weight and she had an intrusive image of herself as an overweight unattractive person that she called 'the repellant drudge'. This worsened her mood and made her more likely to comfort eat. When the image next came to mind, she tried to fast forward to a time where the hard work of dieting and exercising had paid off, and she 'saw' herself at her goal weight doing the things that she'd been able to do before her weight gain. Holding this view of the future in mind gave her hope and motivated her.

Rerunning the image, reviewing and updating it

Sharya wanted to join in college events, but she was unconfident and the thought of being with others was always accompanied by an image of herself lost for words, blushing and feeling unbearably foolish. The emotional impact of this inhibited her. However, she learnt to mentally rerun this image, but she changed the content in line with what she knew about herself, namely she was articulate in class, she was well-informed about current affairs, and she had learnt the art of relaxation. Thus, she was able to change the scene to one where she stood with others, calm and relaxed. She imagined that she was in conversation and engaging others by sharing her perspective on the day's headlines.

When Thom was low he felt lonely and emotionally flat. He sometimes had the image of quietly driving off to a remote layby and taking an overdose. He knew that this was dangerous thinking and he tried to counter it by imagining the drive, but instead he remembered his friendships and imagined his best friend with him touring the countryside, paying attention to the beautiful aspects of the world and reminding himself that he was not alone, that he could feel pleasure, that there was reason to live and that these low periods usually passed.

Devising a new ending so that the story arc of the image is bearable

Di's childhood was unhappy, and she had shadowy memories of being afraid and being hurt. She did not yet want to dwell on those memories, but she did want some relief from them. Her therapist asked her how she felt when these images intruded, and Di reported feeling vulnerable and afraid. Her therapist asked her how she needed to feel in order to cope. Di wanted to feel strong and confident, so her therapist suggested that she consider how the shadowy images might be transformed. Di described imagining herself rising up like a superhero and raising her hand, sending the shadows billowing back. As they disappeared, she saw and felt sunlight and realised that she was standing tall and strong. She felt safe. She rehearsed what she called her 'superhero' scenario and used it each time the shadowy image troubled her. She grew less and less fearful of the dark image and eventually it ceased to bother her. She felt in control.

As with all CBT strategies, distracting and alternative images need to be practised and refined, otherwise they will be less effective in combatting problem images, and of course therapists need to check that imagery techniques are not being used as SSBs. So always review what your patient is learning from the exercise – if the exercise is therapeutic then you should hear that they are enabled by it, not superstitiously clinging to it.

A final note about imagery work – *it should not be undertaken lightly*. Images can be very emotionally evocative, so you should always check that your patient is emotionally robust enough to engage in imagery work. In the examples above, Di was not able to focus on the frightening images per se, that would have overwhelmed her, but she was able to focus on developing a constructive coping scenario. If imagery is particularly traumatic or dangerous in content (e.g. vivid images of harming self or others), then safety needs to be prioritised and breaking confidentiality needs to be considered. An important caution was also raised by Arntz and Weertman in 1999. They advised that therapists working with problem images that appear to be recollections '*must be aware of the (re)constructive processes of memory*' (p. 717). Memory formation and recall is a complex series of processes and it is not infallible. Professor Alan Baddeley's (2004) book, *Your memory: a user's guide*, is an excellent resource for those who need a reminder of the reliability (and unreliability) of memory and the dangers of distorting recollection.

Invaluable generic techniques

There are a number of versatile strategies that are not limited to CBT but which can usefully be incorporated into a CBT approach. Top of my list are assertiveness training and problem solving.

Assertiveness training

Arguably the most fundamental of the social skills, assertiveness lays the foundation for so much of our therapeutic work: anger management, social confidence building, relationship issues, and more. I couldn't do my job without this basic procedure.

In a recent article, Speed, Goldstein and Goldfried (2018) review what they call 'a forgotten evidence-based treatment', reminding us that it has been part of the psychotherapist repertoire since the 1940s. It is recommended by Beck et al. (1979) and has a very persuasive empirical record.

For those who need a refresher on the basics of assertiveness training, the OCTC has a downloadable overview at www.octc.co.uk/wp-content/uploads/2016/10/Assertiveness-OCTC-practical-guide.pdf.

Problem-solving

Problem-solving is a long-established therapeutic technique (D'Zurilla & Goldfried, 1971), particularly in depression (Cuijpers, de Wit, Kleiboer, Karyotaki & Ebert, 2018), and it has been shown to be effective even in a very brief format (Catalan, Gath, Anastasiades & Bond, 1991). Understandably then, Beck and colleagues (1979) remind us that problem-solving is a valuable technique in our CBT toolkit.

Socratic enquiry helps us guide a patient through the stages of:

- defining the problem;
- brainstorming multiple solutions;
- planning to put a solution into action;
- devising contingency plans;
- reviewing the outcome.

Problem-solving has been associated with reduced relapse in several conditions, such as depression (Scott, 2000), obesity (Murawski et al., 2009), and alcohol misuse (Demirbas, Ilhan & Dogan, 2012), so it's worth reviewing a patient's skill prior to discharge.

Again, for those needing a quick refresher, the OCTC has a downloadable document at www.octc.co.uk/wp-content/uploads/2019/11/Problem-Solving-OCTC-practical-guide-.pdf.

While problem-solving is a valuable technique when prompt action is needed, remember that it is always better to plan well in advance if possible. So do discourage patients from putting things off.

Relapse management

Speaking of putting things off, long before discharge a patient should begin learning the skill of relapse management. This is the ability to cope with setbacks by understanding them (i.e. formulating them), learning from them (i.e. reflecting), and moving forward (i.e. problem solving). The term 'management' is often more accurate than 'prevention' as setbacks are common – and even constructive if a person knows how to learn from them.

This is just a brief overview of Relapse Management; a more detailed document can be found on the OCTC website at www.octc.co.uk/wp-content/uploads/2016/07/Relapse-management-2.pdf.

The pioneers of relapse work were Marlatt and Gordon (1985) who developed sophisticated cognitive behavioural methods that are still worth revisiting. However, the essence of relapse management can be captured in three questions that are simple enough to be brought to mind even if someone is distressed:

1. Why is this setback understandable?
2. What have I learnt from it?
3. What will I now do differently?

You can first work through these questions in session, helping your patients learn to decentre and grow familiar with the questions that they can later use in the field.

Jo sometimes binged. One evening she bought quite large quantities of foods and wine, went home alone and consumed most of it. This would usually have marked the beginning of a significant decline. She would have woken the next day in discomfort, would have concluded that she was a hopeless failure and her mood would certainly have been depressed. As a 'hopeless failure' she would have felt powerless to resist the urge to have a numbing glass of wine and/or comfort-eat. However, on this occasion, she decentred and asked:

- *How can I make sense of this lapse?* She appreciated that she'd been stressed at work for several days but had kept pushing on in order not to think about a troubled relationship. In addition, she'd resumed an old habit of starving throughout the day in an attempt to lose weight. Once she had reflected on the situation, she was able to say 'It's no wonder that I fell off the wagon. Not only was I stressed to breaking point, but I also set myself up for a binge by not eating during the day.'
- *What have I learnt from it?* 'For me, it's dangerous to starve as a means of weight control or to try take control of my emotions – it backfires. Also, I need to keep a check on my stress level: when it gets too high, I'm so vulnerable to buying that bottle of wine and comfort-eating.'
- *With hindsight, what will I now do differently?* 'Hard as it is, I would try to eat sensibly during the day without starving. Looking back, I made a mistake in trying to pretend that I did not have problems in my relationship and instead throwing myself into work as a

distraction. If I had that time over again, I would acknowledge my problems, maybe even talk to someone about them rather than ignoring them. I could probably have talked with my brother – he always says that I should. Next time I will.'

This gives Jo more insight into her vulnerabilities as well as a strategy for the future. She will have other setbacks and she can learn from these to refine her personal coping methods.

Relapse management is often enhanced by:

1. *Addressing dichotomous thinking.* People often think in terms of being in *Control* OR *Relapse*. This means that one slip is perceived as failure and then the chance of spiralling into a relapse is high. Better to be able to recognise all the stages en route to actual relapse (see Figure 9.6).

Control	Urge	Setback	Lapse	Relapse

X--X

Figure 9.6

This perspective means that a person is more likely to see a slip or setback as a temporary aberration – one that could be managed.

2. *Being risk sensitive.* Over time people get better at addressing the questions:

    o   'When will I be at risk of this happening?'
    o   'What are the signs?'
    o   'What could I do to avoid losing control?'
    o   'What could I do if I did lose control (damage limitation)?'

In this way 'early warning signs' can be detected, and patients can try to avert trouble, whilst still having a well-considered back-up plan. These headings can form the basis of a *blueprint* (see Chapter 4).

SPECIFIC CBT TECHNIQUES

CBT clinicians and researchers have developed many CBT-specific techniques, and several were introduced in earlier chapters (see Table 9.3).

Table 9.3 Specific CBT techniques

Specific CBT technique	
Thought records	Chapter 7
Data logs	Chapter 7
Downward arrowing	Chapter 7
Responsibility Pie	Chapter 7
Continuum technique	Chapter 7
Worry decision-making tree	Chapter 7
Cost–benefit matrices	Chapter 4
Theory A/Theory B	Chapter 8
Activity schedule	Chapter 8
Graded practice	Chapter 8

Although some strategies were devised to be problem-specific you will find that several are transdiagnostic and thus deserve a place in your basic toolkit.

SUMMARY

- CBT therapists are familiar with a wide range of coping techniques, many of which are transdiagnostic. This enables us to be flexible and respond to patient need.
- Techniques embrace cognitive, behavioural and physical strategies.
- Some are specific within CBT, others are generic within CBT, others are generic across psychotherapies. Our formulations will guide us in best use of strategies.
- By the end of treatment, patients need to know what works for them (the blueprint is a reminder) and how to manage relapse.

REFLECTION & ACTION

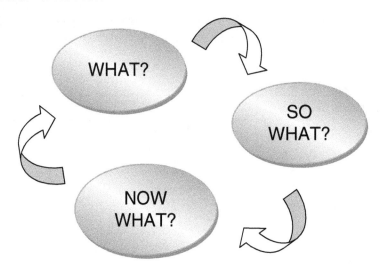

WHAT are you taking away from this chapter? What teaching points resonate with you?

....

....

....

....

....

....

....

....

....

....

SO WHAT? What significance do these points have – how do they relate to your previous learning or views? Do they challenge your former opinions? Have you gleaned new ideas for helping patients or indeed looking after your own needs?

....

....

....

....

....

....

....

....

....

....

NOW WHAT? How will your awareness of your basic tool kit affect your practice? What are you now going to do differently? Make a commitment with yourself to follow through on at least one of your new ideas.

....

....

....

....

....

....

....

....

....

....

10

BUILDING ON THE BASICS: TAKING THINGS FORWARD

Here you are. Familiar with the principles and practice of CBT, but what to do next? I imagine that for most of you reading this book has not been an intellectual exercise; I would guess that you want to continue to develop as a CBT therapist. That's what this chapter is about.

Several years ago, I co-edited a book called *Surviving as a CBT therapist* (Mueller, Kennerley, McManus & Westbrook, 2010). One chapter specifically addressed developing and progressing as a practitioner (McManus, Rosen & Jenkins, 2010). Freda McManus and her co-writers made many good points but one memorable one was that CBT is constantly evolving and so should you. Simple but sound advice. I would recommend reading her chapter, and to holding in mind the guiding notion that a good CBT therapist is one who attends to their development.

DEFINE YOUR GOALS

One of the first recommendations from McManus is be clear about your aims, clarify your targets. Perhaps you want to strive for accreditation, perhaps you want to develop skills in working with a particular clinical population, maybe research interests you. A clear sense of where you want to go will help you structure your continued professional development (CPD) and your evolution as a CBT practitioner.

Joni wanted to become BABCP accredited as a CBT practitioner as soon as possible because her career development depended on this. So she researched the criteria set by the BABCP and created a two-year plan to acquire the relevant training, supervision and practice.

Franklin was a group counsellor with a charity that supported people with brain injury. Now he was more familiar with CBT he hoped to offer CBT to his therapy group members. This meant that he needed to know more about using CBT in groups as well as learning how to adapt CBT for people with cognitive and/or physical impairment.

Mica had worked in a medical research department for several years and more and more she thought that the families of patients would benefit from support, CBT in fact. She wanted to test her hypothesis and her medical director was prepared to fund a small study of CBT family support. Now Mica needed to learn more about using CBT with families and also needed to find a supervisor to guide her.

These examples remind us of the many directions that CBT can take us but there is an overarching principle – we need to be open to more learning.

USE IT, DON'T LOSE IT

It's so well proven that we can't argue with the advice to use it or lose it. There is a tendency toward therapist drift (Waller, 2009) but with regular supervision clinical skills improve (Rako-vshik, McManus, Vasquez-Montes, Muse & Ougrin, 2016) and there is even some evidence that patients benefit (Mannix et al., 2006).

Getting good supervision

So how to ensure you get 'good' supervision? There are registers of accredited CBT supervisors and it is wise to be confident in the credentials of your supervisor and to have a supervision contract that captures your needs. And when you are in supervision, how are you going to make the most of opportunities? One of the most basic things you

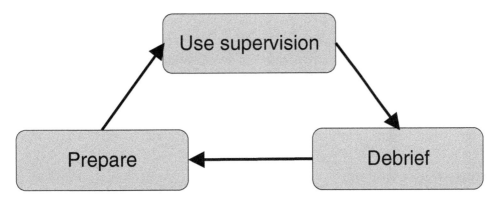

Figure 10.1 Using and preparing for supervision

can do is set aside time for preparing for supervision and for debriefing afterwards (see Figure 10.1).

Preparation

Go into your session having reviewed your caseload, identified your issue(s) for supervision, clarified a clear supervision question(s). Even better, prepare a parsimonious formulation to share with your supervisor. Now you can be focused and economic in your session. You will probably get even more from supervision if you have also identified some excerpts of therapy recordings to illustrate your supervision issue.

During the session

This should be so much more than a discussion – getting the most from time with a supervisor requires structure and attention. Strategies that help us get the most from therapy sessions apply to supervision: setting a mutual and realistic agenda makes best use of time; engaging in role play will help consolidate skills development; incorporating regular mutual feedback will refine learning; attending to the supervisory relationship will ensure the best foundation for meeting supervision needs, and so on. However, do remember that a supervision session is not a therapy session.

Debriefing

After the session take time to debrief and plan: 'What have I learnt? How will I take this forward?' You can invest even more in critical reflection by listening to recordings of your clinical sessions and you can systematically review your performance using instruments such as the ACCS (Muse et al., 2017). This form of self-supervision can be a valuable adjunct to supervision by others.

Other forms of CPD

Don't forget other forms of training: workshops, conferences, books, videos are available to the cognitive therapist. You can even create CPD opportunities by setting up journal clubs in your workplace, for example.

Whatever learning format you choose, the principle of reviewing your experiences and planning how to build on them to create new experiences continues to be relevant to deepening your learning. Keep this in mind.

Use CBT skills to develop and progress as a therapist

As you know, CBT is based on sound psychological principles and as such the strategies and techniques of CBT can help you just as much as they help your patients. We have already talked about setting goals, but what about formulating obstacles when you encounter them, or using your skills of stress management, assertiveness, problem-solving to help you through? It might be worth reviewing your assets and aiming to make the most of them. This will also afford you the opportunity to practise what you preach as a CBT therapist.

Bear in mind McManus's comment that a good CBT practitioner is an evolving practitioner and take stock of your development regularly. If you are progressing in your CBT career, then your strengths and needs will be changing and you will benefit from a regular review. If necessary, make a review date in your diary – that usually helps with remembering and commitment.

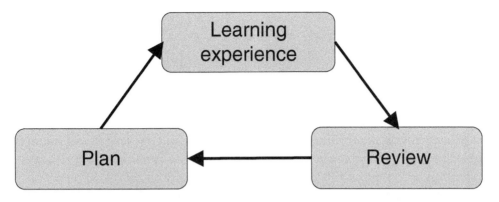

Figure 10.2 Reviewing learning

BE BOLD (BUT NOT RECKLESS)

As you progress, you will meet more clinical challenges. Although we all need to exercise prudent caution, there really is no need to panic when faced with a clinical problem that you've not encountered before, the chances are you can help your patient in some way. A CBT therapist has a very versatile skills set and knowledge base: a formulation framework that is endlessly adaptable to psychological problems and a transdiagnostic toolkit.

Even if you decide that you cannot offer ongoing therapy to a patient with a particular difficulty, you can almost certainly formulate the problem(s) and help them appreciate why their difficulties are understandable. And with a formulation you can begin to explore ideas about alternative interventions: watchful waiting, supportive counselling, self-help, psychodynamic work, couples therapy, family interventions and so on.

In a day dedicated to anxiety, I recently gave a keynote called 'Dissociation: don't panic!'. I was inspired by the many supervisees who retreat at the first inkling of dissociation because of the assumption that it is too challenging a proposition. And there is really no need to retreat because a CBT practitioner has the skills to at least conceptualise a patient's problem, including dissociative problems. I began working with dissociative symptoms in the 1980s when I saw patients with what we would now call C-PTSD and complex trauma. Commonly they would present with flashbacks (a form of compartmentalised dissociation) along with depersonalisation, derealisation, or even out-of-body experiences (forms of detachment dissociation). With nothing but theoretical knowledge of the phenomenon and CBT basics to guide us, patients and I would formulate how the problem presented, what stopped it from remitting, and we might even manage to add an understanding of how the problem came about in the first place. The vicious cycles that we identified guided our intervention. By the 1990s I'd been invited to write a paper on using CBT with dissociative symptoms for the *British*

Journal of Clinical Psychology – and if you can locate such an ancient article, you'll see what I mean about getting a long way with just the basics.

I used the clinical example of dissociation here because I do find that many recoil from it, but really I could have cited any one of the many problems for which we have no well-developed model and protocol as an example of the versatility of the CBT framework and methods.

Having said this, I would not encourage recklessness. If your patient is at risk of harm to self and others your priority is *always* establishing safety, and this might mean not working with them but referring on. If you don't have the theoretical knowledge to support your patient (e.g. younger children or patients who are actively psychotic) then strive to find specialist support or another therapist. Before you use certain techniques check that a patient can tolerate the challenges of using them, e.g. sharing a detailed formulation can engage one person but overwhelm another; using imagery can give swift relief to one patient but be emotionally overstimulating for another; facing a fear rapidly can enhance one person's recovery and yet another person will experience a setback if the pacing is too swift.

Also ask yourself if the patient's system can support and tolerate change, e.g. is your patient able to take enough time away from a needy parent or child to engage fully in CBT at this time? Will your patient be at risk if they are more assertive in their relationship?

A FINAL CONSIDERATION

Colleagues and I recently wrote a paper reflecting on twenty-five years of CBT (Kennerley, Butler, Fennell & Rakovshik, 2020). We looked not only at where we had come from as CBT therapists but also at where we might be heading, and our conclusion was:

> If asked to predict what will happen to CBT over the next quarter century, we would have no hesitation in saying that it will be a survivor, as we continue as we started – with curiosity, humanity and empirical integrity. It has the adaptability, robust theoretical base and empirical foundations to survive. Not without changes, of course, but still recognisable, useful and effective.

This could refer to you – you will survive and grow as a CBT practitioner if you hold on to your genuine curiosity, empathy and empirical stance.

SUMMARY

- Be clear about your objectives for developing as a CBT practitioner.
- Maintain a high quality of ongoing supervision and training.
- Use CBT strategies to enhance your learning and progress.
- Employ reasonable caution but balance this with confidence in the versatility of CBT and the adaptability of your skills base.

FURTHER READING

Kennerley, H., Kirk, J., & Westbrook, D. (2017). *An introduction to cognitive behavior therapy: skills and applications*. London: Sage.

Chapter 19 describes how you can best use CBT supervision.

Mueller, M., Kennerley, H., McManus, F., & Westbrook, D. (2010). *Oxford guide to surviving as a CT therapist*. Oxford: Oxford University Press.

This edited book was aimed at the newly trained CBT therapist, so there is a good chance that you will find it relevant. It covers a lot of ground including, common problems and challenges in practice, working in different specialties, looking after yourself, setting up a private practice, becoming a supervisor and trainer. Chapter 15 specifically describes how you can progress in your CBT career.

Wittington, A., & Grey, N. (2014). *How to become a more effective CBT therapist*. West Sussex: Wiley Blackwell.

Described by one reviewer as 'an invaluable route map for continuing therapist growth and development', this excellent text aims to guide therapists in developing and improving CBT practice. Just what you might be looking for.

REFLECTION & ACTION

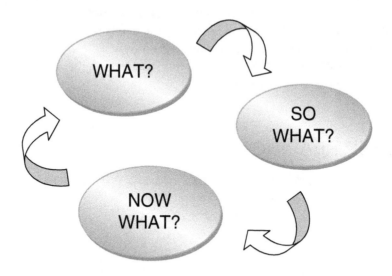

WHAT? You have probably now read the entire text, not just this chapter – what learning points stand out for you?

....

....

....

....

....

....

....

....

....

....

SO WHAT? What strikes you as your best means of taking things forward?

....

....

....

....

....

....

....

....

....

....

NOW WHAT? How are you going to make this happen? Make a plan for moving forward and developing as a CBT practitioner.

....

....

....

....

....

....

....

....

....

....

....

APPENDIX: WORKSHEETS

This section has several useful worksheets – but do remember the value of:

1. *Personalising the worksheet*: use the patient's own language and check that it has validity for them. Discuss the rating scale and make sure that both you and your patient understand what each rating means. Decide what range of rating the patient feels comfortable with, e.g. some people like 1–100 while others find 1–5 works better for them.

2. *Pacing*: don't overwhelm the patient. Sometimes you might introduce part of the worksheet and gradually build on this as your patient becomes more adept at monitoring.

3. *Keeping the endpoint in sight*: monitoring sheets are a means to an end, and that end is usually the skill to stand back and review and revise an automatic response. Make sure that your monitoring activity achieves a meaningful endpoint, and don't fall into the trap of administering something just because you think that's what CBT therapists do!

WORKSHEET 1 – AUTOMATIC THOUGHT RECORD: CATCHING THOUGHTS AND IMAGES

Monitor your feelings and beliefs by rating them using the following scale:

Absent				Moderate				Strong
0	1	2	3	4	5	6	7	8

Date/ Time	EMOTION Rate emotion 0–8	SITUATION What triggered the problem emotion?	AUTOMATIC THOUGHT/IMAGE (COGNITION) Rate belief in this 0–8

WORKSHEET 2 – AUTOMATIC THOUGHT RECORD: CATCHING AND REVIEWING COGNITIONS

Monitor your feelings and beliefs by rating them using the following scale:

Absent				Moderate				Strong
0	1	2	3	4	5	6	7	8

Date/ Time	EMOTION Rate emotion 0–8	SITUATION What triggered the problem emotion?	AUTOMATIC THOUGHT/ IMAGE (COGNITION) Rate belief in this 0–8	IT'S UNDERSTANDABLE THAT I SEE THINGS THIS WAY BECAUSE …	HOWEVER, … What doesn't fit with this view?	NEW CONCLUSION Rating my belief in this new conclusion 0–8	EMOTION Re-rate Emotion 0–8

WORKSHEET 3 – POSITIVE DATA LOG

When you notice one of the following, make a note of it before you forget:

My PDL checklist:

● ....
● ....
● ....
● ....
● ....
● ....
● ....
● ....

0	1	2	3	4	5	6	7	8
Absent				Moderate				Strong

Date/Time	WHAT HAPPENED	WHAT THIS TELLS ME How much I believe this 0–8
What I have learnt about myself over the week:		I believe:

WORKSHEET 4 – BEHAVIOURAL EXPERIMENT RECORD

Rate your beliefs using the following scale:

Absent				Moderate				Strong
0	1	2	3	4	5	6	7	8

Original prediction and belief rating	Specifics of the BE	Outcome	New belief and rating

WORKSHEET 5 – THEORY A/THEORY B RECORD

Event	Evidence for Theory A:	Evidence for Theory B:

Conclusion and what I need to do:

WORKSHEET 6 – ACTIVITY RECORD: MONITORING

Note what you are doing at regular intervals during the day (hourly if possible) and also rate your reactions using the following scale:

Absent		Moderate		Strong
0	1	2	3	4	5

- How ENJOYABLE I found the activity (E: 0–5)
- How meaningful/PURPOSEFUL it seemed (P: 0–5)
- How DIFFICULT it was for me at the time (D: 0–5)

	Monday	Tuesday	Wednesday	Thursday	Friday	Saturday	Sunday
6.00–7.00							
7.00–9.00							
9.00–10.00							
10.00–11.00							
11.00–12.00							
12.00–1.00							
1.00–2.00							
2.00–3.00							
3.00–4.00							
4.00–5.00							
5.00–6.00							
6.00–7.00							
7.00–8.00							
8.00–9.00							
9.00–11.00							
What I've learnt today							

WORKSHEET 7 – ACTIVITY RECORD: PLANNING

Now you have an idea of what helps you feel better, plan your week (hourly if possible) to maximise pleasure and purposefulness.
As your week progresses rate yourself on the following scale:

Absent		Moderate		Strong
0	1	2	3	4	5

- How ENJOYABLE I found the activity (E: 0–5)
- How meaningful/PURPOSEFUL it seemed (P: 0–5)
- How DIFFICULT it was for me at the time (D: 0–5)

	Monday	Tuesday	Wednesday	Thursday	Friday	Saturday	Sunday
6.00–7.00							
7.00–9.00							
9.00–10.00							
10.00–11.00							
11.00–12.00							
12.00–1.00							
1.00–2.00							
2.00–3.00							
3.00–4.00							
4.00–5.00							
5.00–6.00							
6.00–7.00							
7.00–8.00							
8.00–9.00							
9.00–11.00							
What I've learnt today							

WORKSHEET 8 – RELAXATION RECORD

Monitor your progress by rating your level of relaxation before and after carrying out a relaxation exercise. You can use the following scale:

Not relaxed Tense		Moderately relaxed				Very relaxed
0	1	2	3	4	5	6	7	8

Date/ Time	Type of exercise	Rating before	Rating after	Notes

WORKSHEET 9 – COST–BENEFIT MATRIX

Short-term costs	Short-term benefits
Long-term costs	Long-term benefits

My conclusion:

WORKSHEET 10 – BLUEPRINTS

Target: ....

I am at risk when …			
Early warning signs …			
What I can do to stop myself …			
Damage limitation …			

Target: ....

What I've learnt during therapy			
Helpful strategies			
When I'll be at risk of setback			
Ways of responding			

REFERENCES

Arntz, A., & Weertman, A. (1999). Treatment of childhood memories: theory and practice. *Behaviour Research & Therapy, 37*, 715–740.

Barlow, D.H., Hayes, C.H., & Nelson, R.O. (1984). *The scientist practitioner: research and accountability in clinical and educational settings.* Oxford: Pergamon Press.

Barrett, A.M., Crucian, G.P., Schwartz, R.L., & Heilman, K.M. (2000). Testing memory for self-generated items in dementia: method makes a difference. *Neurology, 54*, 1258–1264.

Beck, A.T., Davis, D., & Freeman, A. (2016). *Cognitive therapy of personality disorders* (3rd ed.). New York: Guilford Press.

Beck, A.T., Emery, G., & Greenberg, R.L. (1985). *Anxiety disorders and phobias: a cognitive perspective.* New York: Basic Books.

Beck, A.T., & Haigh, E.A. (2014). Advances in cognitive theory and therapy: the generic cognitive model. *Annual Review of Clinical Psychology, 10*, 1–24.

Beck, A.T., Rush, A.J., Shaw, B.F., & Emery, G. (1979). *Cognitive therapy of depression.* New York: Guilford Press.

Beck, R., & Fernandez, E. (1998). Cognitive-behavioral therapy in the treatment of anger: a meta-analysis. *Cognitive Therapy & Research, 22*, 63–74.

Bennett-Levy, J., Butler, G., Fennell, M., Hackmann, A., Mueller, M., & Westbrook, D. (Eds.). (2004). *The Oxford guide to behavioural experiments in cognitive therapy.* Oxford: Oxford University Press.

Borkovec, T.D., & Newman, M.G. (1999). Worry and generalized anxiety disorder. In P. Salkovskis (Ed.), *Comprehensive clinical psychology, Vol. 6.* Oxford: Elsevier.

Borkovec, T.D., Newman, M.G., Pincus, A.L., & Lytle, R. (2002). A component analysis of cognitive-behavioural therapy for generalized anxiety disorder and the role of interpersonal problems. *Journal of Consulting and Clinical Psychology, 70*(2), 288–298.

Borton, T. (1970). *Reach, touch and teach: student concerns and process education.* New York: McGraw-Hill.

Brown, G.W., & Harris, T.O. (1978). *The social origins of depression: a study of psychiatric disorder in women.* London: Tavistock.

Butler, G., Fennell, M., & Hackmann, A. (2008). *Cognitive behaviour therapy for anxiety disorder: mastering clinical challenges.* London: Guilford Press.

Butler, G., Grey, N., & Hope, T. (2018). *Manage your mind.* Oxford: Oxford University Press.

Catalan, J., Gath, D.H., Anastasiades, P., & Bond, S.A.K. (1991). Evaluation of a brief psychological treatment for emotional disorders in primary care. *Psychological Medicine, 21*, 1013–1018.

Clark, D.M. (1986). A cognitive approach to panic. *Behaviour Research & Therapy, 24*, 461–470.

Clark, D.M. (2002). A cognitive perspective on social phobia. In W.R. Crozier & L.E. Alden (Eds.), *International handbook of social anxiety.* Chichester: Wiley.

Clark, D.M. (2015). Disseminating CBT: science, politics and economics. Keynote presented at the OCTC Congress, Oxford.

Clark, D.M. (2018). Realizing the mass public benefit of evidence-based psychological therapies: the IAPT program. *Annual Review of Clinical Psychology, 14*, 159–183.

Clark, D.M., & Wells, A. (1995). A cognitive model of social phobia. In R. Heimberg, M. Liebowitz, D.A. Hope & F.R. Schneier (Eds.), *Social phobia: diagnosis, assessment and treatment.* New York: Guilford Press.

Cuijpers, P., de Wit, L., Kleiboer, A., Karyotaki, E., & Ebert, D.D. (2018). Problem-solving therapy for adult depression: an updated meta-analysis. *European Psychiatry, 48*, 27–37.

D'Zurilla, T.J., & Goldfried, M.R. (1971). Problem solving and behaviour modification. *Journal of Abnormal Psychology, 78*, 107–126.

Davidson, K., Livingstone, S., McArthur, K., Dickson, L., & Gumley, A. (2007). An integrative complexity analysis of cognitive behaviour therapy sessions for borderline personality disorder. *Psychology and Psychotherapy: Theory, Research and Practice, 80*, 513–523.

Davies, W. (2016). *Overcoming anger and irritability: a self-help guide using cognitive behavioral techniques.* London: Robinson.

Demirbas, H., Ilhan, I.O., & Dogan, Y.B. (2012). Ways of problem solving as predictors of relapse in alcohol dependent male inpatients. *Addictive Behaviors, 37*, 131–134.

Dewey, J. (1933). *How we think: a restatement of the relation of reflective thinking to the educative process.* Boston, MA: D.C. Heath and Company.

Ehlers, A., & Clark, D.M. (2000). A cognitive model of post-traumatic stress disorder. *Behaviour Research & Therapy, 38*, 319–345.

Erdelyi, M., Buschke, H., & Finkelstein, S. (1977). Hypermnesia for Socratic stimuli: the growth of recall for an internally generated memory list abstracted from a series of riddles. *Memory & Cognition, 5*, 283–286.

Fairburn, C.G., Cooper, Z., & Shafran, R. (2003). Cognitive behaviour therapy for eating disorders: a 'transdiagnostic' theory and treatment. *Behaviour Research & Therapy, 41*, 509–528.

Fennell, M. (1999). *Overcoming low self-esteem: a self-help guide using cognitive-behavioural techniques.* London: Constable Robinson.

Fennell, M. (2016). *Overcoming low self-esteem: a self-help guide using cognitive-behavioural techniques* (2nd ed.). London: Constable Robinson.

Garety, P., Kuipers, E., Fowler, D., Freeman, D., & Bebbington, P. (2001). A cognitive model of the positive symptoms of psychosis. *Psychological Medicine, 31*, 189–195.

Gibbs, G. (1988). *Learning by doing: a guide to teaching and learning methods*. London: Further Education Unit.

Gilchrist, P., & Ditto, B. (2012). *Perceived control moderates the vasovagal response*. Poster session presented at 70th Annual Scientific Meeting of the American Psychosomatic Society, Athens, Greece.

Greenberger, D., & Padesky, C. (2016). *Mind over mood* (2nd ed.). New York: Guilford Press.

Hackmann, A., Bennett-Levy, J., & Holmes, E. (2011). *Oxford guide to imagery in cognitive therapy*. Oxford: Oxford University Press.

Harvey, A., Watkins, E., Mansell, W., & Shafran, R. (2004). *Cognitive behavioural processes across psychological disorders: a transdiagnostic approach to research and treatment*. Oxford: Oxford University Press.

Henwood, K.S., Chou, S., & Browne, K.D. (2015). A systematic review and meta-analysis of the effectiveness of CBT informed anger management. *Aggression and Violent Behaviour, 25*, 280–292.

Hofmann, S.G., Asmundson, G.J.G., & Beck, A.T. (2013). The science of cognitive therapy. *Behavior Therapy, 44*, 199–212.

Improving Access to Psychological Therapies (IAPT). Available at: www.england.nhs.uk/mental-health/adults/iapt/

James, I.A., Morse, R., & Howarth, A. (2009). The science and art of asking questions in cognitive therapy. *Behavioural and Cognitive Psychotherapy, 38*, 83–93.

Kazantzis, N., Deane, F., & Ronan, K. (2002). Homework assignments in cognitive and behavioural therapy: a meta-analysis. *Clinical Psychology Science and Practice, 7*, 189–202.

Kennerley, H., Butler, G., Fennell, M., & Rakovshik, S. (2020). *CBT Today, 48*, 20–22.

Kennerley, H., Kirk, J., & Westbrook, D. (2017). *An introduction to cognitive behavior therapy: skills and applications*. London: Sage.

Kirk, J., & Rouf, K. (2004). Specific phobias. In J. Bennett-Levy, G. Butler, M. Fennell, A. Hackmann, M. Mueller & D. Westbrook (Eds.), *Oxford guide to behavioural experiments in cognitive therapy*. Oxford: Oxford University Press.

Kolb, D.A. (1984). *Experiential learning*. New Jersey: Prentice-Hall.

Kuyken, W., Padesky, C.A., & Dudley, R. (2009). *Collaborative case conceptualization: working effectively with clients in cognitive-behavioural therapy*. New York: Guilford Press.

Kvam, S., Lykkedrang Kleppe, C., Nordhus, H.I., & Hovland, A. (2016). Exercise as a treatment for depression: a meta-analysis. *Journal of Affective Disorders, 202*, 67–86.

Layard, R., & Clark, D.M. (2014). *Thrive: the power of psychological therapy*. London: Penguin Books.

REFERENCES

Layden, M., Newman, C., Freeman, A., & Morse, S.B. (1993). *Cognitive therapy of borderline personality disorder.* Boston, MA: Allyn & Bacon.

Lejuez, C.W., Hopko, D.R., Acierno, R., Daughters, S.B., & Pagoto, S.L. (2011). Ten-year revision of the brief behavioral activation treatment for depression: revised treatment manual. *Behaviour Modification, 35,* 111–161.

Lejuez, C.W., Hopko, D.R., & Hopko, S.D.A. (2001). Brief behavioural activation treatment for depression: treatment manual. *Behaviour Modification, 25,* 255–286.

Lewin, K. (1946). *Action research and minority problems. Journal of Social Issues, 2,* 34–46.

Mannix, K., Blackburn, I., Garland, A., Gracie, J., Moorey, S., Reid, B., Standart, S., & Scott, J. (2006). Effectiveness of brief training in cognitive behaviour therapy techniques for palliative care practitioners. *Palliative Medicine, 20,* 579–584.

Mansell, W., Colom, F., & Scott, J. (2005). The nature and treatment of depression in bipolar disorder: a review and implications for future psychological investigation. *Clinical Psychology Review, 25,* 1076–1100.

Marlatt, G.A., & Gordon, J.R. (1985). *Relapse prevention: maintenance strategies in the treatment of addictive disorders.* New York: Guilford Press.

Martell, C.R. (2013). Misconceptions and misunderstandings of behavioural activation: perspectives from a major proponent. *Psychologia, 56,* 131–137.

McManus, F., Rosen, K., & Jenkins, H. (2010). Developing and progressing as a CBT therapist. In M. Mueller, H. Kennerley, F. McManus & D. Westbrook (Eds.), *Oxford guide to surviving as a CT therapist.* Oxford: Oxford University Press.

McMillan, D., & Lee, R. (2010). A systematic review of behavioral experiments vs. exposure alone in the treatment of anxiety disorders: a case of exposure while wearing the emperor's new clothes? *Clinical Psychology Review, 30,* 467–478.

Mikkelsen, K., Stojanovska, L., Polenakovic, M., Bosevski, M., & Apostolopoulos, V. (2017). Exercise and mental health. *Maturitas, 106,* 48–56.

Miller, W.R., & Rollnick, S.R. (2002). *Motivational interviewing: preparing people to change behaviour* (2nd ed.). New York: Guilford Press.

Moorey, S. (2002). *Oxford guide to CBT for people with cancer.* Oxford: Oxford University Press.

Morrison, A. (2001). The interpretation of intrusions in psychosis: an integrative approach to hallucinations and delusions. *Behavioral and Cognitive Psychotherapy, 29,* 247–276.

Mueller, M., Kennerley, H., McManus, F., & Westbrook, D. (2010). *Oxford guide to surviving as a CT therapist.* Oxford: Oxford University Press.

Murawski, M., Milsom, V.A., Ross, K.M., Rickel, K.A., DeBraganza, N., Gibbons, L.M., & Perri, M.G. (2009). Problem solving, treatment adherence, and weight-loss outcome among women participating in lifestyle treatment for obesity. *Eating Behaviour, 10,* 146–151.

Muse, K., & McManus, F. (2013). A systematic review of methods for assessing competence in cognitive-behaviour therapy. *Clinical Psychology Review, 33,* 484–499.

Muse, K., McManus, F., Rakovshik, S., & Thwaites, R. (2017). Development and psychometric evaluation of the Assessment of Core CBT Skills (ACCS): an observation-based tool for assessing cognitive behavioral therapy competence. *Psychological Assessment, 29,* 542–555.

National Institute for Health and Care Excellence (NICE). Available at: www.nice.org.uk/

Novaco, R.W. (1979). The cognitive regulation of anger and stress. In P.C. Kendall & S.D. Hollon (Eds.), *Cognitive-behavioral interventions: theory, research, and procedures.* New York: Academic Press.

Orlinsky, D., Grawe, K., & Parks, B. (1994). Process and outcome in psychotherapy. In A. Bergin & S. Garfield (Eds.), *Handbook of psychotherapy and behaviour change* (4th ed.). New York: Wiley.

Padesky, C. (1994). Schema change processes in cognitive therapy. *Clinical Psychology & Psychotherapy, 1,* 267–278.

Padesky, C. (1996). *Guided discovery using Socratic dialogue* (DVD). Huntington Beach, CA: Center for Cognitive Therapy. Available at: www.padesky.com

Padesky, C., & Greenberger, G. (2020). *The clinician's guide to using Mind over Mood* (2nd ed.). New York: Guilford Press.

Padesky, C.A., & Mooney, K.A. (1990). Clinical tip: presenting the cognitive model to clients. *International Cognitive Therapy Newsletter, 6,* 13–14. (Available from www.padesky.com/clinicalcorner.htm).

Pearson, J., Clifford, C.W.G., & Tong, F. (2008). The functional impact of mental imagery on conscious perception. *Current Biology, 18,* 982–986.

Pretzer, J. (1990). Borderline personality disorder. In A.T. Beck, A. Freeman, D. Davis & associates, *Cognitive therapy of personality disorders.* New York: Guilford Press.

Prochaska, J.O., & DiClemente, C.C. (1986). Towards a comprehensive model of change. In W. Miller & H. Heather (Eds.), *Treating addictive behaviours: processes of change.* New York: Plenum Press.

Rachman, S.J. (2015). The evolution of behaviour therapy and cognitive behaviour therapy. *Behaviour Research and Therapy, 64,* 1–8.

Rakovshik, S.G., McManus, F., Vazquez-Montes, M., Muse, K., & Ougrin, D. (2016). Is supervision necessary? Examining the effects of internet-based CBT training with and without supervision. *Journal of Consulting and Clinical Psychology, 84,* 191–199.

Roth, A., & Fonagy, P. (2005). *What works for whom?* (2nd ed.). New York: Guilford Press.

Roth, A., & Pilling, S. (2007). The competences required to deliver effective cognitive and behavioural therapy for people with depression and with anxiety disorders. London: Department of Health. Document also downloadable from the DoH website archive at: www.dh.gov.uk/prod_consum_dh/groups/dh_digitalassets/@dh/@en/documents/digitalasset/dh_078535.pdf (accessed 13 April 2020).

Rush, A.J., Beck, A.T., Kovacs, M., & Hollon, S.D. (1977). Comparative efficacy of cognitive therapy and pharmacotherapy in the treatment of depressive outpatients. *Cognitive Therapy & Research, 1,* 17–37.

Safran, J.D., & Muran, J.C. (1995). Resolving therapeutic alliance ruptures: diversity and integration. *In Session: Psychotherapy in Practice, 1,* 81–92.

Safran, J.D., & Segal, Z.V. (1990). *Interpersonal process in cognitive therapy.* New York: Basic Books.

Salkovskis, P.M. (1985). Obsessive-compulsive problems: a cognitive-behavioural analysis. *Behaviour Research & Therapy, 23,* 571–583.

Salkovskis, P.M. (Ed.). (1997). *Frontiers of cognitive therapy.* New York: Guilford Press.

Salkovskis, P.M. (1999). Understanding and treating obsessive-compulsive disorders. *Behaviour Research & Therapy, 37,* S29–S52.

Salkovskis, P.M., & Bass, C. (1997). Hypochondriasis. In D.M. Clark & C.G. Fairburn (Eds.), *Science and practice of cognitive-behaviour therapy.* Oxford: Oxford University Press.

Salkovskis, P.M., Clark, D.M., & Gelder, M.G. (1996). Cognitive-behavioural links in the persistence of panic. *Behaviour Research and Therapy, 34,* 453–458.

Salkovskis, P.M., Clark, D.M., Hackmann, A., Wells, A., & Gelder, M.G. (1999). An experimental investigation of the role of safety-seeking behaviours in the maintenance of panic disorder with agoraphobia. *Behaviour Research and Therapy, 37,* 559–574.

Salkovskis, P.M., & Warwick, H.M. (1986). Morbid preoccupations, health anxiety and reassurance: a cognitive-behavioural approach to hypochondriasis. *Behaviour Research & Therapy, 24,* 597–602.

Schmidt, N., & Woolaway-Bickel, K. (2000). The effects of treatment compliance on outcome in cognitive-behavioural therapy for panic disorder: quality versus quantity. *Journal of Consulting and Clinical Psychology, 68,* 13–18.

Scott, J. (1996). The role of cognitive behaviour therapy in bipolar disorder. *Behavioural and Cognitive Psychotherapy, 24,* 195–208.

Scott, J. (2000). Treatment of chronic depression. *New England Journal of Medicine, 342,* 1518–1520.

Segal, Z.V., Williams, J.M.G., & Teasdale, J.D. (2018). *Mindfulness-based cognitive therapy for depression: a new approach to preventing relapse* (2nd ed.). New York: Guilford Press.

Speed, B.C., Goldstein, B.L., & Goldfried, M. (2018). Assertiveness training: a forgotten evidence-based treatment. *Clinical Psychology: Science and Practice, 25,* 1–20.

Szpunar, K.K., & Schacter, D.L. (2013). Get real: effects of repeated simulation and emotion on the perceived plausibility of future experiences. *Journal of Experimental Psychology, 142,* 323–327.

Tarrier, N., & Haddock, G. (2002). Cognitive behavioural therapy for schizophrenia: a case formulation approach. In F.G. Hofmann & M.C. Tompson (Eds.), *Treating chronic and severe mental disorders: a handbook of empirically supported interventions.* New York: Guilford Press.

Teasdale, J.D., Segal, Z., & Williams, M.G. (1995). How does cognitive therapy prevent depressive relapse and why should attentional control (mindfulness) training help? *Behaviour Research and Therapy, 33*, 125–139.

Waller, G. (1993). Why do we diagnose different types of eating disorder? Arguments for a change in research and clinical practice. *Eating Disorders Review, 1*, 74–89.

Waller, G. (2009). Evidence-based treatment and therapist drift. *Behaviour Research and Therapy, 47*, 119–127.

Warwick, H.M.C., & Salkovskis, P.M. (1989). Cognitive and behavioural characteristics of primary hypochondriasis. *Scandinavian Journal of Behaviour Therapy, 18*, 85–92.

Wells, A. (1997). *Cognitive therapy of anxiety disorders: a practice manual and conceptual guide.* Chichester: Wiley.

Wells, A. (2000). *Emotional disorders and metacognition.* Chichester: Wiley.

Wittington, A., & Grey, N. (2014). *How to become a more effective CBT therapist.* West Sussex: Wiley Blackwell.

INDEX